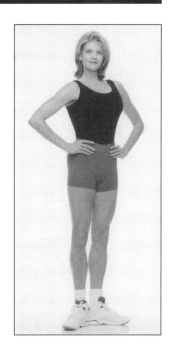

KATHY SMITH'S FITNESS MAKEOVER

A 10-Week Guide to Exercise and Nutrition That Will Change Your Life

Kathy Smith

with Suzanne Schlosberg

WARNER BOOKS

A Time Warner Company

Acknowledgments

My husband, Steve Grace, for his never-ending love and support.
My daughters, Katie and Perrie, for keeping my life in perspective.
Suzanne Schlosberg, my coauthor, for her keen sense of integrity and for always keeping us on track.
My good friends Candace Copeland and Douglas Brooks for their wealth of information and ideas.
Karen Kuchar for her beautifully detailed illustrations.
Marcia Lansdown for her assistance in coordinating this project.
Linda Shelton for her sharp eyesight.

A NOTE FROM THE PUBLISHER
Neither the program in this book, nor any other exercise program, should be followed without first consulting a health care professional. If you have any special conditions requiring attention, you should consult with your health care professional regularly regarding possible modification of the program contained in this book.

Copyright © 1997 by Kathy Smith Enterprises, Inc.
All rights reserved.

Warner Books, Inc., 1271 Avenue of the Americas, New York, NY 10020

Visit our Web site at
http://pathfinder.com/twep

W A Time Warner Company

Printed in the United States of America
First Printing: February 1997
10 9 8 7 6

Library of Congress Cataloging-in-Publication Data
Smith, Kathy.
    [Fitness makeover]
    Kathy Smith's fitness makeover : a 10-week guide to exercise
and nutrition that will change your life / Kathy Smith.
        p.   cm.
    Includes index.
    ISBN 0-446-67049-9
    1. Exercise. 2. Nutrition. 3. Physical Fitness. 4. Weight loss.
I. Title
RA781.S613   1997
613.7—dc20
                                        96-5550
                                          CIP

Book design by H. Roberts
Cover design by Diane Luger
Cover photo by Michael Greco

Contents

Introduction

Congratulations! With this book in hand, you're on your way to creating that lean, firm, healthy body you've always wanted. I admire anyone willing to take on this challenge, anyone ready to take responsibility for their own health and fitness. It's easy to sit there and complain about being flabby, unmotivated, or hooked on junk food; it's a lot tougher to actually do something about it.

Now, I realize that making major lifestyle changes can seem pretty overwhelming. All of a sudden, you're supposed to eat less fat and more fiber, consume less sugar and more calcium, drink less soda and more water, and on and on. At the same time, you want to reduce your hips, firm up your arms, and tighten your bottom! But let's be honest: You just can't do everything at once. You could pull it off for a week or two, but soon you'd start feeling deprived of your old, familiar habits, and you'd feel yanked in a million directions. Eventually, you'd probably want to run from it all and just plop down on the couch with the remote control.

That, of course, isn't the answer. In this book, you'll discover a much better one. After twenty-five years working hard to improve my own health and fitness, I've concluded that success comes down to one word: focus. The one surefire strategy is to *focus* your energy on one single healthy habit at a time—to learn why that particular habit is so important and practice adapting it to your own tastes and preferences. After a while, you'll incorporate that new healthy habit into your life without extra effort. It'll just become second nature! Once you conquer one goal— whether it's cutting back on saturated fat or strengthening your abdominals—you'll be inspired to tackle another, and another. It's like a domino effect. But a good one. Before you know it, you'll have generated enough momentum to carry you through a complete transformation of your exercise and eating habits.

The Focus Plan

My ten-week program is based entirely on the focus concept. It contains everything you need to get fit and lose weight, including:

- a low-fat eating strategy that's practical and easy to follow
- effective muscle-toning workouts to target your whole body in 20 to 30 minutes
- a simple, calorie-burning cardiovascular exercise plan

Throughout the program you'll be performing total-body workouts, but each week you'll *focus* on a particular body area, such as your thighs, buttocks, or shoulders. The same principle applies to the eating plan. Every week you'll strive to eat a low-fat, balanced diet, but you'll also *focus* on one special nutrition goal, such as cutting back on saturated fat or eating more fiber. Ten weeks from now, you'll look back and see how much your habits have changed—and you'll be amazed at what a smooth, easy transition it's been.

The Program: Keeping a Log

Perhaps the most critical component of my program—the tool that'll make it all come together—is the daily log. Think about it: Doesn't it help to be able to *see* what you're focusing on? In this book, you'll see your goals printed on paper. Every day you'll take a few minutes to record your workouts and food choices. Then, at the end of the week, you'll tally up your accomplishments, turn the page, and start focusing on your new goals for the week ahead.

Why bother with all this record keeping? That's an easy one to answer: Nothing will inspire you more than seeing your own triumphs in writing. It's documented proof of all your hard work! When you meet your goals at the end of the week, you'll want to keep your streak going—to keep knocking down those dominoes. At the end of 10 weeks, you'll flip back through your log and say, "Wow, I did all *that?*" It'll only motivate you to do more.

Learning from Your Log

Your log will also give you tremendous insight into your own habits. We all say, "I should eat less fat." But do you have any idea how much fat you're eating *now?* We all say, "I should work out more." But do you have any idea how many calories you've burned while exercising this week? Your log will enable you to pinpoint exactly where you need to concentrate your efforts. Maybe you're consistent with your toning workouts, but you're letting your cardiovascular exercise slide. Maybe your fat intake is just fine, but you're eating too many calories. In order to make appropriate changes in your habits, you first need to know what your habits *are!*

You might be surprised by what you learn. I sure was. I'm always preaching to my friends about the importance of calcium. Well, during the 10 weeks we all tested out my log, I found out *I* was the one short on calcium! It seemed like I was eating a cup of yogurt every day, but in fact I was only having it three or four times a week. Now yogurt is my regular afternoon snack.

I no longer keep a log every day of my life, but it's a tool I often turn to when my weight starts creeping up. It's quite a wakeup call! Sometimes, I get into a phase where I grab a handful of walnuts every time I walk by the fridge. When I'm forced to record this in my diary, I say, "My gosh! That's 33 grams of fat—nearly my entire daily fat budget—and it wasn't even a planned snack." Your log will make you aware of your "sub-snacks," the foods you don't even realize you're eating. We all have ways of fooling ourselves; we convince ourselves that if we don't look at the package, those cookies *can't* be loaded with fat! Whether you're eating too much fat, skimping on fiber, or neglecting to exercise, your log will hold you accountable.

A Friend for the Duration

Consider this book your companion for the next 10 weeks. It'll be there for you every day—guiding you through your workouts, encouraging you to choose healthy foods, and steering you back on track when you start to veer off in the wrong direction. It'll help you *focus* on concrete, realistic goals. And most important, it'll guarantee that for all the effort you put in, you'll get the credit you deserve.

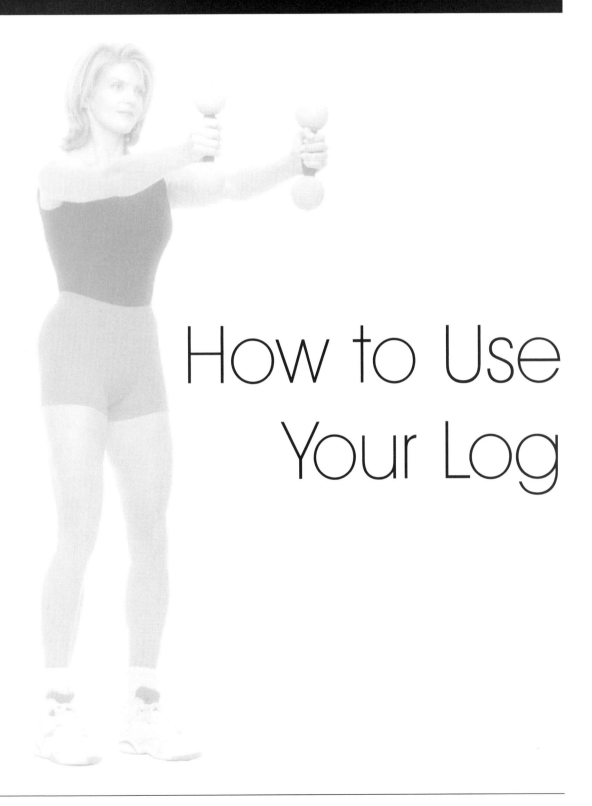

Part 1

How to Use Your Log

o let's get going! Your log has four key components: Toning, Cardio Exercise, Stretching, and Nutrition. Over the next 10 weeks, I'll provide you with specific goals in all four of these areas. Your mission is to work hard at fulfilling the goals and to record your progress in your daily log. I've designed the log so it's easy to use—you'll get the hang of it after just a few days.

Here's a step-by-step look at how to follow the program and fill in each section of the log.

The Weekly Plan

At the beginning of each week, you'll find a one-page list of your exercise and nutrition goals. This is a summary of your assignments for the week. It's broken down into four parts: Toning Goals, Toning Routine, Cardio Goals, and Nutrition Goals.

Toning Goals

At the top of the page is a box that describes the week's toning goals. Here, for instance, is the plan for Week 1:

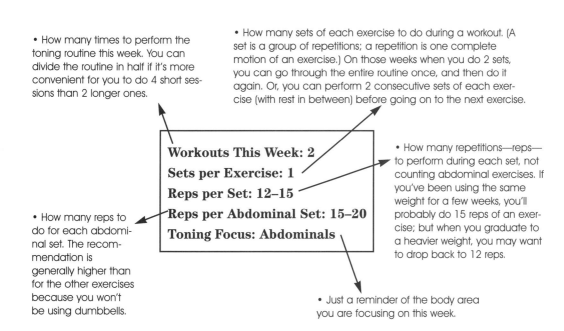

• How many times to perform the toning routine this week. You can divide the routine in half if it's more convenient for you to do 4 short sessions than 2 longer ones.

• How many sets of each exercise to do during a workout. (A set is a group of repetitions; a repetition is one complete motion of an exercise.) On those weeks when you do 2 sets, you can go through the entire routine once, and then do it again. Or, you can perform 2 consecutive sets of each exercise (with rest in between) before going on to the next exercise.

Workouts This Week: 2
Sets per Exercise: 1
Reps per Set: 12–15
Reps per Abdominal Set: 15–20
Toning Focus: Abdominals

• How many repetitions—reps—to perform during each set, not counting abdominal exercises. If you've been using the same weight for a few weeks, you'll probably do 15 reps of an exercise; but when you graduate to a heavier weight, you may want to drop back to 12 reps.

• How many reps to do for each abdominal set. The recommendation is generally higher than for the other exercises because you won't be using dumbbells.

• Just a reminder of the body area you are focusing on this week.

Toning Routine

The next part of the weekly plan is a chart listing the week's exercises and the reference page for each exercise description and photo. In order to do the workouts, you'll need three sets of dumbbells—light (1 to 3 pounds), medium (3 to 5 pounds), and heavy (10 to 15 pounds). Ankle weights are optional, and if you are familiar with how to use exercise tubing or bands, you can use them to make the exercises tougher.

Every routine works your entire body in 12 exercises, but they're never the *same* 12. For instance, in Week 1, your chest exercise is the Push-up; in Week 2, it's the Chest Flye. Each workout begins with the Focus exercises, which are shaded.

TONING EXERCISE	PAGE
1. Reverse Curl	212
2. Crunch	210
3. Cross Crunch	214
4. Push-up	238

Cardio Goals

Next comes the week's plan for cardiovascular exercise—crucial for burning fat and strengthening your heart and lungs. Here's what Week 1 looks like:

Cardio Exercise
Calories to Burn: 350+
Total Days: 3+

Each week, you have two cardio goals: a minimum number of *calories* to burn and a minimum number of *days* to work out. In Week 1, for instance, your goal is to burn at least 350 calories during the week and do aerobic exercise on at least 3 days. You can choose to burn about 115 calories over 3 days, 70 calories over 5 days—or any other configuration you'd like. It's all up to you, as long as you meet the minimum requirement. To estimate how many calories you burn, use the chart on pages 12–13. You can choose any activity you want, such as walking, swimming, cycling, step aerobics, in-line skating. Just make sure it's fun!

Also, be sure to exercise at a moderate intensity. When you're working out, you should always be able to talk. It's okay if you have to take a few breaths between sentences, but if you're so worn out that you can't utter two consecutive words, slow down. If you're chatting as easily as you do on the telephone, speed up.

Throughout the program, your Cardio Goal increases by 50 calories per week. This isn't much at all—it means walking just an extra half mile per *week*. I encourage you to exceed my minimum recommendation. If you want to lose weight—not just improve your health—you will want to burn extra calories. (See Week 3's discussion of Calories, on page 57, for more details on how to lose weight.)

Nutrition Goals

At the bottom of the Weekly Plan page, I'll remind you of the week's Food Focus and the specific food goal. The details of how to achieve this goal will be explained in the week's food discussion. Week 1 looks like this:

> **Food Focus:** Fat
> **Goal:** Count fat grams; become aware of your fat intake

The Toning Pages

After the Weekly Plan you'll find three identical Toning pages. Each one has your week's routine already written in, with the Focus exercises shaded. All you have to do is fill in the number of sets and reps you did and the amount of weight you lifted. For instance, let's say you did 1 set of 15 reps for each of the abdominal exercises, 1 set of 8 push-ups, then 1 set of 12 squats with a 5-pound dumbbell in each hand. Here's what you'd write:

	SETS	REPS	WEIGHT
1. Reverse Curl	1	15	—
2. Crunch	1	15	—
3. Cross Crunch	1	15	—
4. Push-up	1	8	—
5. Squat	1	12	5

Although you never *need* to do more than two toning workouts per week, there will always be an optional third toning page to accommodate those of you who want to work out with weights three days a week. You fill in the days of the week. Be sure to rest at least 48 hours between toning sessions.

The Daily Log

Here's where you'll record everything *other* than toning: Cardio Exercise, Stretching, and Nutrition. You have a full page for each day of the week, plus a special Week in Review page to tally up your accomplishments.

Cardio Exercise

If you jogged for 15 minutes, then walked for another 15, you might fill in the cardiovascular exercise section like this:

CARDIO EXERCISE	TIME	CALORIES BURNED
JOG 15, WALK 15	30	240

• In the first box, describe your activity. You might want to include details such as how you felt ("step class—tough!"), how far you went ("swam 30 laps"), who you exercised with ("walked with Laura"), what type of terrain you covered ("cycled Pig Farm Hill"), or how the weather treated you ("walked; hot and humid!").

• In the second box jot down how many minutes you worked out. If you took three 10-minute walks, you might want to write "10 + 10 + 10" rather than "30." This will give you more insight into your exercise patterns.

• Third, use the chart on pages 12–13 to estimate how many calories you burned during your cardio workout.

Stretching

This section is simple: Just check off whether or not you stretched:

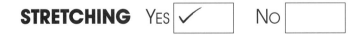

STRETCHING   YES ✓   NO

I recommend stretching every day—you can do my entire stretching routine in 5 to 10 minutes! (See Stretches, page 199.) You can stretch whenever you want; just make sure you warm up first with at least 5 minutes of light aerobic exercise. Hold each position for 10 to 60 seconds, stretching to the point of mild tension, but not pain. Always use slow, controlled movements. Never bounce or bob up and down.

Nutrition

Over the course of my program, you'll work on developing a truly balanced diet—one that's both *low in fat* and *high in nutrients*. Each day you'll keep track of your progress on both fronts by 1) counting your fat grams and 2) monitoring your food-group servings. Let's use Week 1 as an example.

NUTRITION Fat Budget _38_ grams	**Fat Grams**
Breakfast: low-fat Yoplait berry yogurt, 6 oz 8 am 1 banana, 2 oz Grape Nuts 6 oz orange juice	3g
Snack: 1 apple 10:30 1 Tbsp peanut butter	8g

• Each morning, fill in your daily Fat Budget—the number of fat grams you ideally want to consume during the day. My Fat Budget is 38 grams; to find yours, see "Your Fat Budget," page 10. You can "spend" your fat grams however you'd like, but spend them wisely. If you know there's an office birthday party at lunch, plan ahead by eating an extra-low-fat breakfast, so that you can "bank" some fat grams for the cake. You're bound to exceed your Fat Budget on some days—that's okay. Just don't make it a habit. At the same time, don't let banking your fat grams turn into a cycle of depriving yourself and then bingeing.

• In the spaces provided, record everything you eat during the day. I mean *everything!* Be specific about the amounts *and* the type of food. Write "1 1/2 cups brown rice" instead of just "rice." Write "6 oz. strawberry nonfat yogurt" instead of just "yogurt." Make your notes just after you eat; it's so easy to forget how much dressing you poured on your salad or how many potato chips you ate.

• Notice that I've given you just as much space to jot down your snacks as I have for breakfast, lunch, and dinner. Research suggests that eating four or five small meals per day may be more effective for weight control than eating three large ones. Keeping track of snacking can help those who eat too much throughout the day to be aware of how much extra they're eating. If you eat small portions every few hours, you'll avoid becoming ravenously hungry, which is often what leads to overeating. The chart is designed to encourage frequent, small meals.

• In addition to listing your food choices, you might also want to record the *time* of your meal or snack. If, for instance, you're always starving by lunchtime, your log may help you understand why; maybe you ate breakfast at 7:30 A.M. and didn't eat again until 1 P.M.

• Consider jotting down your thoughts and feelings about eating. Were you truly hungry for your snack, or did you just eat it out of habit? Did you really want that ice cream or did you raid the freezer out of boredom?

• In the shaded Fat Grams column on the right-hand side of the chart, add up your fat grams for each meal, then tally up the totals at the bottom. You'll need one of those small books that list the fat and calorie content for nearly every food you can think of, such as *The Fat Counter* (Pocket Books) or *Brand Name Fat and Cholesterol Counter* (American Heart Association). You can buy one in any bookstore for $5 to $10. I recommend choosing one that also includes grams of saturated fat, which is the Food Focus for Week 2.

• In the Notes box, you can size up your day overall. Try to write something positive! Maybe you met your Fat Budget for the first time, or maybe you snacked on yogurt with fruit instead of your usual Snickers bar. Don't wait until you've lost 10 pounds to congratulate yourself. Give yourself credit for the small victories, too. Remember, your ultimate goal is to change your lifestyle, not just fit into your jeans.

YOUR FAT BUDGET

The United States Department of Agriculture recommends that we get no more than 30 percent of our calories from fat. However, I don't think we should settle for the government's goal. For optimal health, many experts prefer a diet closer to 20 percent fat. This translates into a certain number of fat grams per day—your Fat Budget. To figure out the magic number for you, first find your Ideal Weight using the charts on the next page. (The numbers are based on an appropriate calorie intake, which, in turn, is an *estimate* based on your height and frame size. Your individual calorie needs will also be greatly affected by the amount of muscle you have; the more muscle you have, the more energy you need.)

IDEAL WEIGHT

WOMEN

Height Feet	Inches	Small Frame	Medium Frame	Large Frame
4	10	102–111	109–121	118–131
4	11	103–113	111–123	120–134
5	0	104–115	113–126	122–137
5	1	106–118	115–129	125–140
5	2	108–121	118–132	128–143
5	3	111–124	121–135	131–147
5	4	114–127	124–138	134–151
5	5	117–130	127–141	137–155
5	6	120–133	130–144	140–159
5	7	123–136	133–147	143–163
5	8	126–139	136–150	146–167
5	9	129–142	139–153	149–170
5	10	132–145	142–156	152–173
5	11	135–148	145–159	155–176
6	0	138–151	148–162	158–179

MEN

Height Feet	Inches	Small Frame	Medium Frame	Large Frame
5	2	123–134	131–141	138–150
5	3	130–136	133–143	140–153
5	4	132–138	135–145	142–156
5	5	134–140	137–148	144–160
5	6	136–142	139–151	146–164
5	7	138–145	142–154	149–168
5	8	140–148	145–157	152–172
5	9	142–151	148–160	155–176
5	10	144–154	151–163	158–180
5	11	146–157	154–166	161–184
6	0	149–160	157–170	164–188
6	1	152–164	160–174	168–192
6	2	155–168	164–178	172–197
6	3	158–172	167–182	176–202
6	4	162–176	171–187	181–207

Source: Metropolitan Life Insurance Company.

Now that you've located your Ideal Weight, use the next chart to find your Fat Budget.

FAT BUDGET

IDEAL WEIGHT	FAT BUDGET
90	26
100	28
110	30
120	34
130	36
140	40
150	44
160	48
170	52
180	56
190	60
200	62
210	66
220	68

Food Group Servings

These days nutrition experts have moved beyond the four food groups concept that many of us grew up with. The system in my program has six food groups. At the bottom of each log page you'll find the following chart:

FOOD GROUP SERVINGS

Fruits	○ ○ ○ ○ ○
Vegetables	○ ○ ○ ○
Calcium-Rich	○ ○ ○
Protein-Rich	○ ○ ○ ○
Breads/Grains	○ ○ ○ ○ ○ ○ ○ ○
Water	○ ○ ○ ○ ○ ○ ○ ○

Your goal isn't necessarily to check off *every* box. The chart below will help you determine the number of servings *you* need from each food group. Refer to the Fat Budget chart first, then find the number of servings that match up. For instance, if your Fat Budget is 32 grams, you'll aim for 3 vegetable servings, 2 fruit servings, and so on. To learn what constitutes a serving, see "Serving Sizes," page 11.

DAILY FOOD GROUP SERVINGS

FAT BUDGET	FRUITS	VEGETABLES	CALCIUM-RICH	PROTEIN-RICH	BREADS/GRAINS	WATER
26–28g	2	2	2	2	5	8
30–34	2	3	2	3	6	8
36–40	3	3	2	3	7	8
46–50	4	4	3	3	8	8
52+	5	4	3	4	9	8

If you consume the recommended number of daily servings for each group, you can enjoy a satisfying, wholesome, high-energy diet. But remember: These are just guidelines; the details are up to you. Sure, a slice of white bread counts as a bread serving, but it's not as nutritious as a slice of whole wheat. Three-fourths of a cup of apple juice counts as a fruit serving, but it doesn't have the nutrient density of a plain apple.

SERVING SIZES

Let's take a look at what exactly constitutes a serving.

Fruits

- 1 piece medium-sized fruit
- 1/2 cup chopped, cooked, or canned fruit
- 3/4 to 1 cup raw fruit
- 3/4 cup fruit juice
- 1/4 cup raisins or other dried fruit

Vegetables

- 1 cup of raw, leafy vegetables
- 1/2 cup of other veggies, cooked or chopped raw
- 1 medium potato
- 3/4 cup vegetable juice

Calcium-Rich

- 1 cup milk or yogurt
- 1½ ounces natural cheese
- 2 ounces processed cheese
- 1/2 cup ricotta cheese
- 1 cup tofu

Protein-Rich

- 2–3 ounces of cooked meat, poultry, or fish
- 1/2 cup cottage cheese
- 1 cup cooked beans
- 1 cup tofu
- 2 eggs or 3 egg whites
- 4 tablespoons peanut butter or 1/2 cup nuts or seeds (note: high in fat)
- 2 ounces cheese

Breads/Grains

- 1 ounce cereal, bread, bagel, roll, crackers, tortilla
- 1/2 cup cooked rice, pasta, cereal
- 3 cups air-popped or light popcorn

Water

- 1 cup (8 ounces) of water, sparkling water, or mineral water

(You can get plenty of water through juices, sodas, and other drinks, but most of these choices add calories and sugar. Plain water is the best choice.)

Week in Review

At the end of each week, there's a page devoted to recapping your exercise and nutrition accomplishments of the week. It's important to take a step back and look at the big picture. This will give you a more accurate sense of your progress. It's not catastrophic if you skip your aerobics class one day or eat two slices of pie with dinner. But if you're consistently doing it, you need to work harder at improving your lifestyle. The Week in Review will keep you honest; it forces you to compare your actual accomplishments with what you set out to do. All it takes is a few simple tallies:

- Toning: Note how many days you did your toning routine and whether or not you met the Toning Goal.
- Cardio Exercise: Record how many days you worked out, how many calories you burned, and whether or not you met the cardio goals.
- Weight: Don't weigh yourself more than once a week, and make sure you use the same scale at the same time of day.
- Nutrition: Indicate how many days you met your Fat Budget. For the Food Focus goal, rate your progress on a scale of 1 to 5 (5 being best).

CALORIES BURNED

Use this chart to *estimate* how many calories you burn while exercising. The numbers are based on a 130-pound woman; a 180-pound man will burn about 30 percent more. Keep in mind that the number of calories you burn depends on your weight, muscle mass, and metabolism, as well as the intensity of your workout. In general, a moderate workout of any kind will burn 4 to 5 calories per minute; a highly fit person who really cranks up the intensity can burn 10 to 12 calories per minute.

ACTIVITY	15 MINUTES	30	45	60
Aerobics (high-impact)	104	207	311	414
Aerobics (low-impact)	74	148	222	296
Ballet	89	177	266	354
Bicycling (12 to 14 mph)	118	236	354	472
Box aerobics	133	265	398	530
Circuit weight training	118	236	354	472
Cross-country skiing	150	300	450	600
Downhill skiing	74	148	222	296
Golf (carrying clubs)	81	162	243	324
In-line skating	104	207	311	414
Jumping rope (moderate)	148	295	443	590
Karate, tae kwon do	148	295	443	590
Kayaking	74	148	222	296

ACTIVITY	15 MINUTES	30	45	60
Mountain biking	126	251	377	502
Racquetball	104	207	311	414
Rowing machine	150	300	450	600
Running (8.5 minute mile)	170	339	509	678
Ski machine	140	280	320	560
Slide (moderate)	101	201	302	402
Stairclimber	105	210	315	420
Stationary biking (vigorous)	155	310	465	620
Step aerobics	169	337	506	674
Swimming (crawl, 50 yards per minute)	143	285	428	570
Tai chi	59	118	177	236
Tennis (singles)	118	236	354	472
VersaClimber	161	322	483	644
Walking (12-minute mile)	113	225	413	550
(15-minute mile, flat)	88	175	263	350
(20-minute mile, flat)	63	125	188	250
(20-minute mile, 4% incline)	100	200	300	400
Water aerobics	59	118	177	236
Weight lifting (vigorous)	89	177	266	354
Yoga	59	118	177	236

ILLUSTRATIONS OF MAJOR MUSCLE GROUPS

Here are illustrations of your body's major muscle groups. Refer to them when you read each week's "Muscle Basics" discussion. The diagrams are another tool to help you focus on the muscle group of the week.

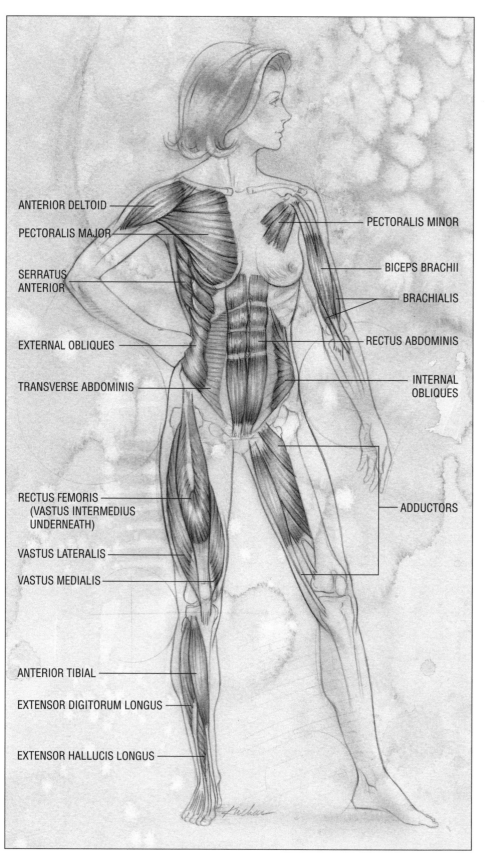

ANTERIOR DELTOID

PECTORALIS MAJOR

SERRATUS ANTERIOR

EXTERNAL OBLIQUES

TRANSVERSE ABDOMINIS

RECTUS FEMORIS (VASTUS INTERMEDIUS UNDERNEATH)

VASTUS LATERALIS

VASTUS MEDIALIS

ANTERIOR TIBIAL

EXTENSOR DIGITORUM LONGUS

EXTENSOR HALLUCIS LONGUS

PECTORALIS MINOR

BICEPS BRACHII

BRACHIALIS

RECTUS ABDOMINIS

INTERNAL OBLIQUES

ADDUCTORS

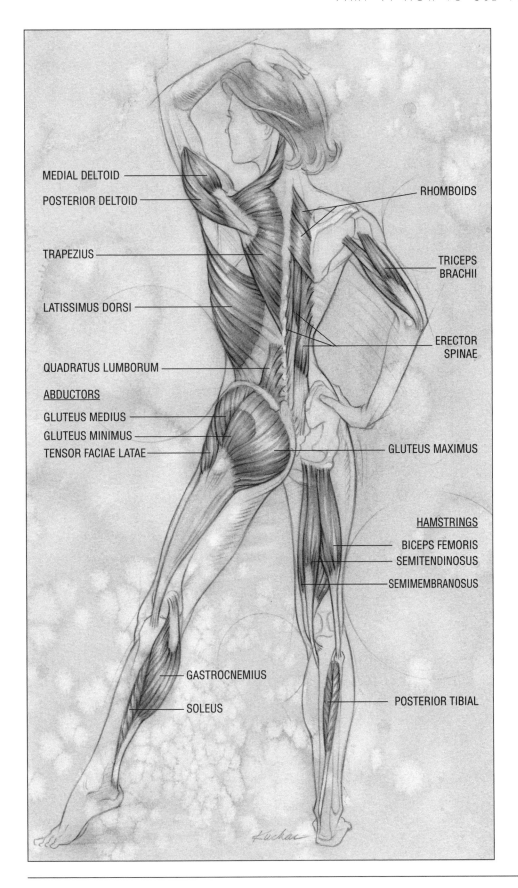

MEDIAL DELTOID

POSTERIOR DELTOID

TRAPEZIUS

LATISSIMUS DORSI

QUADRATUS LUMBORUM

ABDUCTORS

GLUTEUS MEDIUS

GLUTEUS MINIMUS

TENSOR FACIAE LATAE

GASTROCNEMIUS

SOLEUS

RHOMBOIDS

TRICEPS BRACHII

ERECTOR SPINAE

GLUTEUS MAXIMUS

HAMSTRINGS

BICEPS FEMORIS

SEMITENDINOSUS

SEMIMEMBRANOSUS

POSTERIOR TIBIAL

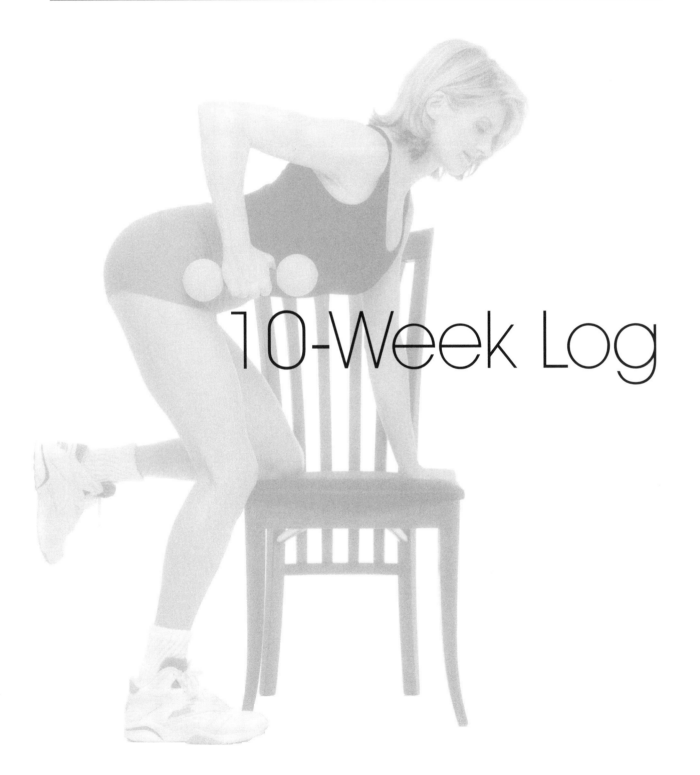

Part II

10-Week Log

FAT AND ABS

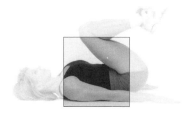

Fat

NUTRITION GOAL RECAP

Use this week to become aware of your fat intake—not to slash it. Eat the way you normally do and count your fat grams. You have the next 9 weeks to work on meeting your Fat Budget.

Time for a quick quiz. Which has more fat:
- A Nutri-Grain blueberry cereal bar or three Duncan Hines chocolate chip cookies?
- A Burger King Fish Filet Sandwich or a McDonald's Quarter Pounder with Cheese?

Granola bars and fish sound a lot leaner than cookies and hamburgers, but in these cases—and plenty of others—they have even *more* fat. That's why it's crucial to scrutinize labels and learn about the fat content of restaurant foods. Sure, we've all gotten the cut-the-fat message, but studies show we often don't know how to put our knowledge into action. SnackWell's fat-free cookies may be flying off the shelves, but Americans are still eating way too much fat.

Over the course of this program, you'll aim for a diet that's 20 percent fat. But this week, your goal is to become *aware* of fat—not to slash it. Eat the way you normally do and count your fat grams. Don't panic if you're way over your Fat Budget. The U.S. government isn't going to solve *its* budget crisis overnight; neither are you. It's not a smart approach, anyway. Studies show that making instant, radical changes in fat intake only sets you up for a rebound effect of fat bingeing.

Still, cutting extra fat out of your diet is a lot easier than it seems. You don't need to deprive yourself; you just need to train your body to judiciously choose when and how much fat to eat. After a while, you will actually *prefer* grilled chicken to fried chicken, strawberry sorbet to strawberry ice cream. Research shows the gradual approach works. In one six-month study, subjects reported that the longer they remained on a low-fat diet, the more they began to dislike the creamy, greasy taste of fatty foods. More than 60 percent said they actually felt physical discomfort after eating high-fat foods. I've experienced this myself. When I see potato salad drenched in mayonnaise, it turns my stomach. Meanwhile, I've gained a great appreciation for the flavor of fresh foods. Trust me—eventually you won't feel like drowning your veggies in butter!

We're all creatures of habit—we stick with the foods we enjoy. So, rather than go on some crazy diet program, learn to lighten up your regular meals. If you love tuna sandwiches, replace mayonnaise with something less fattening. For me, plain nonfat yogurt has been a saving grace. I combine it with Dijon mustard, add a little soy, and toss in a few herbs. I get the moistness of mayo but none of the fat. Searching for tricks like this makes low-fat eating an adventure!

Dropping from a 40 percent fat diet to a 20 percent fat diet sounds like a tall order, but you can accomplish your goal by making subtle changes. Look at these two breakfast menus.

The 40 percent fat version:
　　2 pieces toast
　　2 fried eggs
　　1/2 tablespoon butter
　　1 tablespoon jam
　　1 cup melon
　　1 cup coffee with 1 teaspoon sugar

The 20 percent fat version:
　　2 pieces toast
　　1 fried egg
　　2 ounces lean ham
　　1 tablespoon jam
　　1 1/2 cups melon
　　1 cup coffee with 1 teaspoon sugar

Abs

I have a confession to make: Abdominal exercises aren't number one on my list of favorite fitness activities. It's not terribly exciting to lie on your back and stare at the ceiling. But I'll tell you what has kept me motivated: results. I'm not talking about the washboard abs promised on magazine covers—"5 Minutes To A Flat Tummy" and "A Flat Belly Right Now!" No, I'm a realist. And I'm talking about the firm, sexy middle that comes from exercising your abs consistently.

You don't need to do hundreds of crunches; a few dozen performed properly will do the trick. I usually start my workouts with ab exercises because I want to give them extra-special concentration. After having two kids, my abs have been stretched and stretched and stretched! It takes a lot of work to tighten them back up. (And even then, you can't expect to completely regain your original muscle tone.)

Ab exercises aren't going to melt away fat around your middle, but they can make you *look* 10 pounds lighter. How? By improving your posture. If you have an overarched back, for instance, your bottom might stick out and appear larger than it really is. Abdominal exercises will help you stand up straight and walk with a tall, graceful posture. They'll also make your everyday life easier. You use your abs every time you carry groceries, sit at your computer, even stand in line at the movies. The stronger your abs, the more likely you'll be able to ward off lower back pain.

A final word on abs: Many people are obsessed with developing that flat-as-a-board look. But the truth is, our abdominal muscles are just not designed to be perfectly flat. It's natural for many women to have a slight bulge in the abdomen. Work hard to strengthen your middle, but don't worry yourself over that small curve below your belly button. As long as it's toned, it's sexy!

Muscle Basics

You have four abdominal muscles. The largest is the *rectus abdominis,* which runs straight down your torso. You use this muscle when you bend forward and sideways. Although you often hear people refer to the "upper abs" and "lower abs," the rectus abdominis is really one muscle. However, you can perform exercises that favor one portion or the other.

Your waist muscles are your *external* and *internal obliques.* They help you twist, bend sideways, or bend forward. Your deepest abdominal muscle is the *transverse abdominis,* which wraps horizontally around your torso and helps hold your internal organs in place. You don't need to do exercises that specifically target this muscle; it gets worked when you tone the other abdominal muscles.

Week 1: The Plan

Workouts This Week: 2
Sets per Exercise: 1
Reps per Set: 12–15
Reps per Abdominal Set: 15–20
Toning Focus: Abdominals

TONING EXERCISE	PAGE
1. Reverse Curl	212
2. Crunch	210
3. Cross Crunch	214
4. Push-up	238
5. Squat	226
6. Back Extension	216
7. Seated Back Flye	236
8. Standing Side Lift	228
9. Lateral Raise	242
10. Standing Calf Raise	256
11. French Press	248
12. Seated Biceps Curl	252

Cardio Exercise
Calories to Burn: 350+
Total Days: 3+

Food Focus: Fat
Goal: Count fat grams; become aware of your fat intake

TONING DAY 1

DATE ___6/7/2004___

FOCUS: **Abdominals**

	SETS	REPS	WEIGHT
1. Reverse Curl	1	20	Ø
2. Crunch	1	20	Ø
3. Cross Crunch	1	20 each side	Ø
4. Push-up	1	15	ø
5. Squat	1	15	ø
6. Back Extension	1	15	Ø
7. Seated Back Flye	1	15	ø
8. Standing Side Lift	1	15 each	ø
9. Lateral Raise	1	15	ø
10. Standing Calf Raise	1	15	Ø
11. French Press	1	15	ø
12. Seated Biceps Curl	1	15	ø

TONING DAY 2

DATE _____

Focus: **Abdominals**

	SETS	REPS	WEIGHT
1. Reverse Curl			
2. Crunch			
3. Cross Crunch			
4. Push-up			
5. Squat			
6. Back Extension			
7. Seated Back Flye			
8. Standing Side Lift			
9. Lateral Raise			
10. Standing Calf Raise			
11. French Press			
12. Seated Biceps Curl			

TONING DAY 3

DATE _____

FOCUS: **Abdominals**

	SETS	REPS	WEIGHT
1. Reverse Curl			
2. Crunch			
3. Cross Crunch			
4. Push-up			
5. Squat			
6. Back Extension			
7. Seated Back Flye			
8. Standing Side Lift			
9. Lateral Raise			
10. Standing Calf Raise			
11. French Press			
12. Seated Biceps Curl			

Week 1 MONDAY DATE _6/7/2004_

CARDIO EXERCISE | TIME | CALORIES BURNED
_414_

STRETCHING YES [×] No [ ]

_Aerobic class
1 hour_

NUTRITION FAT BUDGET _35_ GRAMS

FAT GRAMS

Breakfast: _Milk 1 glass_ _Blueberies_ _1 piece of white bread_ _1 cup of black coffee_	
Snack: _1 glass of water_ _yougurt low fat_	
Lunch: _soup (tomatos + pasta)_ _2 crocers_	
Snack: _1 glass of cherries_	
Dinner: _2 cottlets_ _1 glass of water_ _1/2 califlower (steamer)_ _1 glass cocacola 1glass of juice_	
Notes:	**Totals:**

FOOD GROUP SERVINGS

Fruits ◐◐◐○○○
Vegetables ◐○○○
Calcium-Rich ◐◐○
Protein-Rich ◐○○○
Breads/Grains ◐○○○○○○○○○
Water ◐◐○○○○○○○

Food Fact

Recent research suggests that high-fat intake is not linked to breast cancer. However, the issue is far from settled. Countries with high-fat diets have high rates of breast cancer, and scientists are searching for answers to explain why.

For your serving goals, refer to page 11.

Week 1 TUESDAY   DATE [ ]

CARDIO EXERCISE   TIME   CALORIES BURNED

[ ]   [ ]   [ ]

STRETCHING   YES [ ]   NO [ ]

NUTRITION   FAT BUDGET _____ GRAMS

		FAT GRAMS
Breakfast:	glass of milk with oat meal black coffee	
Snack:	yogurt lowfat	
Lunch:	½ cauliflower (steamed) 1 glass off cooked grikai	
Snack:	glass of water	
Dinner:	cutlet green salad 2 glasses of water 1 glass juice 1 glass tea	
Notes:		**Totals:**

FOOD GROUP SERVINGS

2 Fruits   ○ ○ ○ ○ ○
3 Vegetables   ○ ○ ○ ○
2 Calcium-Rich   ○ ○ ○
5 Protein-Rich   ○ ○ ○ ○
7 Breads/Grains   ○ ○ ○ ○ ○ ○ ○ ○ ○
8 Water   ○ ○ ○ ○ ○ ○ ○ ○ ○

𝕵ood 𝕵act

Your body needs some fat to function. Fat is essential for absorbing vitamins A, D, E, and K; maintaining your immune system; and keeping your skin moist. It also helps you feel satisfied longer. If you consistently eat less than 20 percent fat, you may get hungry before you have the opportunity to eat again.

For your serving goals, refer to page 11.

Week 1 WEDNESDAY DATE

CARDIO EXERCISE | TIME | CALORIES BURNED

STRETCHING YES ☐ No ☐

NUTRITION FAT BUDGET _____ GRAMS

FAT GRAMS

	FAT GRAMS
Breakfast: *slice of black bread* *small piece of smoked salmon* *black coffee*	
Snack: *1 banana*	
Lunch: *coffee* *cooked grilled 1 glass*	
Snack: *1 bananas*	
Dinner: *spicy chicken wings* *½ cup* *slice of black bread* *greenpiece* *small piece of smoked salmon*	
Notes:	**Totals:**

FOOD GROUP SERVINGS

Fruits ◐ ◐ ◯ ◐ ◯
Vegetables ◐ ◯ ◯ ◯
Calcium-Rich ◯ ◯ ◯
Protein-Rich ◐ ◯ ◯ ◯
Breads/Grains ◐ ◐ ◯ ◐ ◯ ◯ ◯ ◯
Water ◐ ◐ ◐ ◐ ◯ ◯ ◯ ◯

Fitness Tip

It may take some trial and error to determine how heavy your dumbbells should be. You know you have the right weight if your last two reps of a set are difficult, but you're still able to maintain proper form. If you get to your 15th rep and feel like you could easily do a few more, your weight is too light.

For your serving goals, refer to page 11.

Week 1 THURSDAY DATE ____

CARDIO EXERCISE | TIME | CALORIES BURNED
____ | ____ | ____

STRETCHING YES ____ NO ____

NUTRITION FAT BUDGET ____ GRAMS

	FAT GRAMS
Breakfast: Milk (glass) with cereal / black coffee	
Snack: 1 water	
Lunch: french fries / fried beef / coce (glass)	
Snack: glass water / 8 strawberries	
Dinner: glass of milk with cereal / 1/2 banana / sandwich: 2 slices of whole bread, sandwich turkey, 1 tomato, letuce	
Notes:	**Totals:**

FOOD GROUP SERVINGS

Fruits ◉◉○○○○
Vegetables ◉◉○○
Calcium-Rich ◉◉○
Protein-Rich ○○○○
Breads/Grains ◉◉◉○○○○○○○
Water ◉◉○○○○○○○

Food Fact

"Low-fat" 2 percent milk doesn't get 2 percent of its calories from fat—it gets 38 percent. The 2 percent refers to the amount of *weight* that comes from fat. Whole milk is 51 percent fat, 1 percent milk is 20 percent fat, and skim milk is 4 percent fat.

For your serving goals, refer to page 11.

Week 1 FRIDAY   DATE [   ]

CARDIO EXERCISE   TIME   CALORIES BURNED
[   ]   [   ]   [   ]

STRETCHING YES [   ]   NO [   ]

NUTRITION FAT BUDGET _____ GRAMS   FAT GRAMS

	FAT GRAMS
Breakfast: *black coffee*	
Snack: *peach water 1 glass*	
Lunch: *clam chowder soup*	
Snack: *Bananas*	
Dinner:	
Notes: **Totals:**	

FOOD GROUP SERVINGS

Fruits   ◐ ◐ ○ ○ ○ ○
Vegetables   ○ ○ ○ ○
Calcium-Rich   ○ ○ ○
Protein-Rich   ◐ ○ ○ ○
Breads/Grains   ○ ○ ○ ○ ○ ○ ○ ○ ○
Water   ◐ ◐ ◐ ◐ ◐ ○ ○ ○

Fitness Tip

Have a friend take a full-body picture of you and paste it someplace visible, such as on your refrigerator. Ten weeks from now, take another picture, and you'll see just how far you've come. No doubt you'll look healthier, slimmer, more toned, and more energetic!

For your serving goals, refer to page 11.

Week 1 SATURDAY   DATE [ ]

CARDIO EXERCISE   TIME   CALORIES BURNED

[ ]   [ ]   [ ]

STRETCHING YES [ ]   NO [ ]

NUTRITION FAT BUDGET _____ GRAMS

	FAT GRAMS
Breakfast:	
Snack:	
Lunch:	
Snack:	
Dinner:	
Notes: **Totals:**	

FOOD GROUP SERVINGS

Fruits   ○ ○ ○ ○ ○
Vegetables   ○ ○ ○ ○
Calcium-Rich   ○ ○ ○
Protein-Rich   ○ ○ ○ ○
Breads/Grains   ○ ○ ○ ○ ○ ○ ○ ○ ○
Water   ○ ○ ○ ○ ○ ○ ○ ○

Food Fact

Low-fat eating may help prevent skin cancer. One study showed that nonmelanoma skin cancer sufferers who cut fat from 40 percent to 20 percent of total calories developed one-third the number of precancerous lesions as those who continued eating 40 percent fat.

For your serving goals, refer to page 11.

Week 1 SUNDAY   DATE

CARDIO EXERCISE   TIME   CALORIES BURNED

STRETCHING   YES ☐   NO ☐

NUTRITION   FAT BUDGET _____ GRAMS

FAT GRAMS

	FAT GRAMS
Breakfast:	
Snack:	
Lunch:	
Snack:	
Dinner:	
Notes: **Totals:**	

FOOD GROUP SERVINGS

Fruits   ○ ○ ○ ○ ○
Vegetables   ○ ○ ○ ○
Calcium-Rich   ○ ○ ○
Protein-Rich   ○ ○ ○ ○
Breads/Grains   ○ ○ ○ ○ ○ ○ ○ ○ ○
Water   ○ ○ ○ ○ ○ ○ ○ ○

Food Fact

Late-night fat cravings are most common when you skip meals and when you eat too much sugar during the day. The more often you snack on fatty foods at night, the more likely you'll crave those snacks in the future.

For your serving goals, refer to page 11.

WEEK IN REVIEW

TONING

DAYS [ ]   DID YOU MEET THE GOAL? _____

NOTES _____

_____

CARDIO EXERCISE

DAYS [ ]   CALORIES [ ]   DID YOU MEET THE GOALS? _____

NOTES _____

_____

WEIGHT [ ]

NUTRITION

DAYS UNDER FAT BUDGET [ ]   FOOD FOCUS RATING, 1–5 [ ]

You're off to a great start!

Remember: Everyone who has ever taken a big step has been afraid at the beginning.

Kathy

SATURATED FAT
AND LOWER BACK

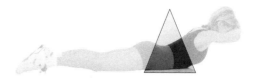

Saturated Fat

NUTRITION GOAL RECAP

This week, aim to meet your Saturated Fat Budget. To determine this number, cut your Fat Budget in half. To fill in your log, you'll need a fat-counting book that includes saturated fat grams, such as The Fat Counter (Pocket Books) or Brand Name Fat and Cholesterol Counter (American Heart Association).

Now that you're a pro at counting fat grams, it's time to take a more sophisticated look at your fat intake. This week's lesson: All fats are not created equal. They all have 9 calories per gram, and they're all easily converted into body fat. But they can have radically different effects on your health.

Saturated fat can cause the most damage, raising your blood cholesterol level and increasing your risk for heart disease. Experts say it's not enough to keep your overall fat intake down. You also need to keep your saturated fat intake low—to less than 10 percent of your calories. Studies show that people of the Mediterranean region have far lower incidences of heart disease and diet-influenced cancers than we do, even though their diets average up to 40 percent fat. This is thought to be because they get just 8 percent of their calories from *saturated* fat.

This week, in addition to counting fat grams (as you will for the rest of the program), you'll count saturated fat grams. Determine your daily Saturated Fat Budget by cutting your Fat Budget in half. My Fat Budget is 38 grams, so my Saturated Fat Budget is 19 grams. To fill in your log this week, you'll need a fat-gram book that also includes saturated fat grams.

Before we take a close look at the different types of fat, let's clear up some confusion about cholesterol. People often think that cholesterol is a type of fat. But in fact it's a substance that has no calories and is found only in animal products, such as beef, poultry, fish, cheese, eggs, and milk. Eating foods high in cholesterol may raise the level of cholesterol in your blood, but eating saturated fats will raise your blood cholesterol far more.

Once inside your body, cholesterol combines with other substances to form lipoproteins. There are two types of lipoproteins: LDLs (*low*-density lipoproteins, nicknamed the "bad cholesterol") and HDLs (*high*-density lipoproteins, the "good cholesterol"). If you have too many LDLs, they start sticking to the walls of your arteries, gradually choking off the flow of blood. HDLs, meanwhile, act as vacuum cleaners within your bloodstream, helping to remove the bad lipoproteins from your body. The higher your HDL level, the lower your risk of developing heart disease. It's hard to remember which type of cholesterol is which, so here's a trick I use: You want your "high" to go higher and your "low" to go lower.

Now let's consider how different types of fat affect your cholesterol levels. Keep in mind that foods generally contain mixtures of saturated and unsaturated fats, with one type of fat predominating.

• *Saturated Fats.* They're found primarily in meats such as beef, pork, and ham, and in dairy products such as whole milk, ice cream, and cheese. Saturated fats increase LDLs, which can lead to clogged arteries, heart attacks, and strokes.

• *Polyunsaturated Fats.* Found mostly in corn, soybean, safflower, and sunflower oils, these fats have been shown to increase levels of HDLs, the good cholesterol.

• *Monounsaturated Fats.* Found mostly in vegetable and nut oils, such as olive, peanut, and canola, they seem to reduce LDL levels without affecting HDLs. However, the impact appears to be modest.

• *Trans Fatty Acids (TFAs).* These fats are created when polyunsaturated oils are chemically altered through hydrogenation, a process used to turn liquid vegetable oils into solids like margarine and shortening. Hydrogenation keeps baked goods fresh longer, but research suggests that TFAs act like saturated fats, raising LDL levels and increasing heart disease risk. These fats compose up to 60 percent of the fat in processed foods such as Ritz Crackers and Pop Tarts. Labels don't tell you about trans fatty acids; try to avoid foods that contain "hydrogenated vegetable oil."

BUTTER OR MARGARINE?

Which is better? Margarine wins because it's lower in saturated fat. But stick to liquid or whipped margarines, which contain fewer trans fatty acids than stick margarines. The best are those with water or a liquid vegetable oil listed as the first ingredient. Next best: those that start off with "vegetable oil blend," a combination of liquid and partially hydrogenated oils. If the label lists "partially hydrogenated oil," don't buy it. Another tip: Ideally, margarine should contain twice as much polyunsaturated fat as saturated fat. The bottom line is, try to keep your added fats to a minimum, and unless you *need* the harder fats—in cooking, for instance—try to stick to liquid fats.

Lower Back

If there's one area of the body most of us overlook, it's the lower back. Naturally, we focus on toning the muscles we can see—our abs, legs, arms, chest, and shoulders. People don't go around saying, "Hey, you've got a *terrific* lower back." But in reality, no muscle group deserves more attention.

Think of your body as a house. Long before you start decorating, you've got to build a strong foundation; otherwise the structure will cave in. The foundation for your body's strength comes from your abdominal and lower back muscles. If they're weak, your body isn't going to hold up. At that point, the decorating—sculpted arms and shoulders, for instance— won't matter.

There's no telling when lower back pain will strike. You're especially prone if you spend a lot of time sitting at a desk or driving a car. In those positions, your lower back muscles tend to stretch out. If ignored, they'll eventually weaken. However, if you commit to a few simple lower back exercises, you'll feel a remarkable sense of confidence in your body. You'll trust it to be there for you, whether you're moving furniture, carrying an overloaded laundry basket, or doing the squats and lunges in my workout program. I get a kick out of the fact that I can change the 10-gallon jug in my water cooler at the house! And I'll tell you, the best feeling in the world is to go for a hike and throw your kid on your back with ease. That beats a "great legs" compliment any day.

Muscle Basics

The muscles of your lower back are your *erector spinae* and your *quadratus lumborum*. These muscles help hold your body in an upright position, and they pull you back up from a bent-over position.

Week 2: The Plan

Workouts This Week: 2
Sets per Exercise: 1
Reps per Set: 12–15
Reps per Abdominal Set: 15–20
Toning Focus: Lower Back

TONING EXERCISE	PAGE
1. Back Extension	216
2. Back Extension with a Twist	218
3. Chest Flye	240
4. Backward Lunge	222
5. Cross Crunch	214
6. One-Arm Row	234
7. Inner Thigh Pull	230
8. Concentration Curl	254
9. Hamstring Curl	232
10. Triceps Kickback	250
11. Toe Raise	258
12. Front Raise	244

Cardio Exercise
Calories to Burn: 400+
Total Days: 3+

Food Focus: Saturated Fat
Goal: Meet your Saturated Fat Budget

TONING DAY 1

DATE _____

FOCUS: **Lower Back**

	SETS	REPS	WEIGHT
1. Back Extension			
2. Back Ext. with Twist			
3. Chest Flye			
4. Backward Lunge			
5. Cross Crunch			
6. One-Arm Row			
7. Inner Thigh Pull			
8. Concentration Curl			
9. Hamstring Curl			
10. Triceps Kickback			
11. Toe Raise			
12. Front Raise			

TONING DAY 2

DATE _____

FOCUS: **Lower Back**

	SETS	REPS	WEIGHT
1. Back Extension			
2. Back Ext. with Twist			
3. Chest Flye			
4. Backward Lunge			
5. Cross Crunch			
6. One-Arm Row			
7. Inner Thigh Pull			
8. Concentration Curl			
9. Hamstring Curl			
10. Triceps Kickback			
11. Toe Raise			
12. Front Raise			

TONING DAY 3

DATE _____

FOCUS: **Lower Back**

	SETS	REPS	WEIGHT
1. Back Extension			
2. Back Ext. with Twist			
3. Chest Flye			
4. Backward Lunge			
5. Cross Crunch			
6. One-Arm Row			
7. Inner Thigh Pull			
8. Concentration Curl			
9. Hamstring Curl			
10. Triceps Kickback			
11. Toe Raise			
12. Front Raise			

Week 2 MONDAY   DATE [ ]

CARDIO EXERCISE   TIME   CALORIES BURNED

[ ]   [ ]   [ ]

STRETCHING   YES [ ]   NO [ ]

NUTRITION   FAT BUDGET _____   SATURATED FAT BUDGET _____

	FAT GRAMS	SATURATED FAT GRAMS
Breakfast:		
Snack:		
Lunch:		
Snack:		
Dinner:		
Notes: **Totals:**		

FOOD GROUP SERVINGS

Fruits   ○ ○ ○ ○ ○
Vegetables   ○ ○ ○ ○
Calcium-Rich   ○ ○ ○
Protein-Rich   ○ ○ ○ ○
Breads/Grains   ○ ○ ○ ○ ○ ○ ○ ○ ○
Water   ○ ○ ○ ○ ○ ○ ○ ○

Food Fact

When your doctor checks your blood cholesterol, ask to see your LDL/HDL breakdown. Low risk for heart disease is associated with LDL levels lower than 130 mg per 100 ml, HDLs 35 or higher, and total cholesterol less than 200.

Week 2 TUESDAY   DATE [ ]

CARDIO EXERCISE   TIME   CALORIES BURNED

[ ]   [ ]   [ ]

STRETCHING YES [ ]   NO [ ]

NUTRITION FAT BUDGET _____   SATURATED FAT BUDGET _____

	FAT GRAMS	SATURATED FAT GRAMS
Breakfast:		
Snack:		
Lunch:		
Snack:		
Dinner:		
Notes: **Totals:**		

FOOD GROUP SERVINGS

Fruits   ○ ○ ○ ○ ○
Vegetables   ○ ○ ○ ○
Calcium-Rich ○ ○ ○
Protein-Rich ○ ○ ○ ○
Breads/Grains ○ ○ ○ ○ ○ ○ ○ ○ ○
Water   ○ ○ ○ ○ ○ ○ ○ ○

Food Fact

Olive oil, like other monounsaturated fats, has been shown to raise HDL levels and reduce the risk of heart disease. But remember: Olive oil should be enjoyed in place of, not in addition to, other fats like butter and margarine.

Week 2 WEDNESDAY DATE

CARDIO EXERCISE | TIME | CALORIES BURNED

STRETCHING YES ☐ NO ☐

NUTRITION FAT BUDGET _____ SATURATED FAT BUDGET _____

	FAT GRAMS	SATURATED FAT GRAMS
Breakfast:		
Snack:		
Lunch:		
Snack:		
Dinner:		
Notes: **Totals:**		

FOOD GROUP SERVINGS

Fruits ○ ○ ○ ○ ○
Vegetables ○ ○ ○ ○
Calcium-Rich ○ ○ ○
Protein-Rich ○ ○ ○ ○
Breads/Grains ○ ○ ○ ○ ○ ○ ○ ○
Water ○ ○ ○ ○ ○ ○ ○ ○ ○

Fitness Tip

Before your toning workouts, warm up with a 5- to 10-minute walk or other cardio activity. Arm circles will help get your blood pumping through your upper body. Remember: Warm muscles are less likely to get injured than cold ones.

Week 2 THURSDAY DATE

CARDIO EXERCISE TIME CALORIES BURNED

STRETCHING YES NO

NUTRITION FAT BUDGET _____ SATURATED FAT BUDGET _____

	FAT GRAMS	SATURATED FAT GRAMS
Breakfast:		
Snack:		
Lunch:		
Snack:		
Dinner:		
Notes: **Totals:**		

FOOD GROUP SERVINGS

Fruits   ○ ○ ○ ○ ○
Vegetables   ○ ○ ○ ○
Calcium-Rich   ○ ○ ○
Protein-Rich   ○ ○ ○ ○
Breads/Grains   ○ ○ ○ ○ ○ ○ ○ ○ ○
Water   ○ ○ ○ ○ ○ ○ ○ ○ ○

Food Fact

An 8-gram daily reduction of saturated fat could reduce U.S. health care costs by as much as $17 billion a year. The savings would come from a 36 percent drop in coronary artery disease, which costs the country $48 billion annually.

Week 2 FRIDAY   DATE [   ]

CARDIO EXERCISE   TIME   CALORIES BURNED
[   ]   [   ]   [   ]

STRETCHING YES [   ]   NO [   ]

NUTRITION FAT BUDGET _____   SATURATED FAT BUDGET _____

	FAT GRAMS	SATURATED FAT GRAMS
Breakfast:		
Snack:		
Lunch:		
Snack:		
Dinner:		
Notes: Totals:		

FOOD GROUP SERVINGS

Fruits	○ ○ ○ ○ ○
Vegetables	○ ○ ○ ○
Calcium-Rich	○ ○ ○
Protein-Rich	○ ○ ○ ○
Breads/Grains	○ ○ ○ ○ ○ ○ ○ ○ ○
Water	○ ○ ○ ○ ○ ○ ○ ○ ○

Fitness Tip

Lift your dumbbells slowly. Swinging your weights will generate momentum and make the exercise too easy on your muscles. Pause at the top of the motion to let your muscles fully contract. Remain in control on both the lifting *and* return phase of each repetition.

Week 2 SATURDAY   DATE _____

CARDIO EXERCISE   TIME   CALORIES BURNED

STRETCHING   YES _____   NO _____

NUTRITION   FAT BUDGET _____   SATURATED FAT BUDGET _____

	FAT GRAMS	SATURATED FAT GRAMS
Breakfast:		
Snack:		
Lunch:		
Snack:		
Dinner:		
Notes: **Totals:**		

FOOD GROUP SERVINGS

Fruits   ○ ○ ○ ○ ○
Vegetables   ○ ○ ○ ○
Calcium-Rich   ○ ○ ○
Protein-Rich   ○ ○ ○ ○
Breads/Grains   ○ ○ ○ ○ ○ ○ ○ ○ ○
Water   ○ ○ ○ ○ ○ ○ ○ ○

Food Fact

A Belgian waffle with whipped cream has almost twice as much saturated fat as biscuits and gravy and as much saturated fat as two McDonald's Quarter Pounders, according to the Center for Science in the Public Interest.

Week 2 SUNDAY

DATE

CARDIO EXERCISE

TIME

CALORIES BURNED

STRETCHING YES NO

NUTRITION FAT BUDGET _____ SATURATED FAT BUDGET _____

	FAT GRAMS	SATURATED FAT GRAMS
Breakfast:		
Snack:		
Lunch:		
Snack:		
Dinner:		
Notes:	**Totals:**	

FOOD GROUP SERVINGS

Fruits ○ ○ ○ ○ ○
Vegetables ○ ○ ○ ○
Calcium-Rich ○ ○ ○
Protein-Rich ○ ○ ○ ○
Breads/Grains ○ ○ ○ ○ ○ ○ ○ ○ ○
Water ○ ○ ○ ○ ○ ○ ○ ○

Food Fact

Trans fatty acids may cause 30,000 heart disease deaths each year. In one study, women with the highest intake of trans fatty acids (6 grams per day) were 50 percent more likely to develop heart disease than those who ate less than half as much.

WEEK IN REVIEW

TONING

DAYS [ ]   DID YOU MEET THE GOAL? _____

NOTES _____

_____

CARDIO EXERCISE

DAYS [ ] CALORIES [ ]   DID YOU MEET THE GOALS? _____

NOTES _____

_____

WEIGHT [ ]

NUTRITION

DAYS UNDER FAT BUDGET [ ]   FOOD FOCUS RATING, 1–5 [ ]

Don't just focus on reaching your end goals. The real success lies in taking control and making it happen right now.

Kathy

CALORIES
AND BUTTOCKS

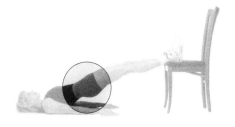

Calories

NUTRITION GOAL RECAP

This week your goal is to meet your Calorie Budget, based on the chart below.

Even though the spotlight these days is on fat, you shouldn't forget about calories. The bottom line is, if you consume too many of them—whether they're from fat, carbohydrate, or protein—you'll gain weight. And if you eat fewer calories than you expend, you'll *lose* pounds!

This week you'll do some good old-fashioned calorie counting. First, find your Calorie Budget in the chart below. (To find your Ideal Weight, refer to the charts on page 9, which you used to determine your Fat Budget.)

CALORIE BUDGET

IDEAL WEIGHT	CALORIE BUDGET
90	1170
100	1260
110	1350
120	1530
130	1620
140	1800
150	2070
160	2250
170	2340
180	2520
190	2700
200	2790
210	2970
220	3060

Keep in mind, these are only *estimates;* your actual budget depends on your metabolism, your activity level, and your goals. This chart assumes you're just starting an exercise program, and it reflects the approximate number of calories you need to maintain your current weight. To *lose* weight, cut back a bit on the calories you eat while increasing the number of calories you burn. (If you cut back by drastically restricting your calorie intake, your body will sense that it is being starved and will fight back by slowing down your metabolism—that is, burning fewer calories.)

Be patient with weight loss. It takes a deficit of 3,500 calories to lose a pound of body fat. In order to lose a pound a week, you need an average daily deficit of 500 calories. You could accomplish this by burning 250 calories through exercise (doing a 45-minute aerobic video, for instance) and eating 250 calories less than normal (a 2-egg omelette with 2 ounces of cheese instead of a 3-egg omelette with 3 ounces of cheese). Keep in mind that burning 250 calories a day through exercise requires a much bigger commitment than the minimum goal in my program.

This week, use your fat-gram book to log in calories. If you discover you're going over budget on a low-fat diet, you're not alone. Nutritionists say something unexpected has happened since Americans started paying attention to fat: People have gained even *more* weight. For some people, the Four Food Groups are Entenmann's, Healthy Choice, Lean Cuisine, and SnackWell's! Don't confuse the term "low-fat" with "low-calorie." If a food is "fat-free," you can't just eat unlimited amounts without any consequences; plenty of fat-free and low-fat foods are high in calories. Some low-fat ice creams have nearly the same number of calories as their high-fat counterparts—they're just loaded with extra sugar!

Getting extra calories from sugary foods is just one problem. Ironically, I've found that it's easy to get too many calories from wholesome, nutritious foods, too. It's because they're so good! If I'm on a business trip where I'm confronted with greasy, high-fat foods, it's easy to stick to small portions because the food isn't appealing to me. It's only when I come home that I'm prone to overeating. I just love pasta primavera with broccoli, carrots, asparagus tips, and mushrooms. It's so delicious that I pile it on my plate—and that's when my weight starts creeping up. You really *can* get too much of a good thing. Ultimately, when it comes to deciding how much to eat, don't simply count calories; pay close attention to how your body *feels*. Often, you'll be satisfied with a lot less food than you think.

Buttocks

If you're looking for a boost from behind—and who isn't?—the key word is overload. The muscles of your rear end have plenty of endurance, since you put them to use whenever you walk. But if you really want to shape, tone, and lift your bottom, endurance isn't going to cut it. You need to focus on strength. This is something I've learned from years of experience. I used to have a somewhat flabby rear end, but I've worked hard to change it. You can, too.

I always look forward to my buttocks routine. The moves aren't easy—they require a fair amount of balance and coordination—but I'm always up for the challenge. Most of my exercises do more than just strengthen the glutes (your buttocks and hip muscles); they also involve the rear thigh muscles and sometimes the front thigh muscles, too. It's important to do multi-muscle exercises like these because, in real life, your muscles work together as an integrated unit. It's not often that you'd be down on all fours lifting one leg in the air, as you are in some glutes-only exercises.

And speaking of real life: With strong buttocks muscles, you'll bound past your co-workers climbing the stairs at the office, and you'll have no trouble chasing your kids up a hill. If you're into sports, powerful glutes will give you extra oomph when you jump up to shoot a basket or spike a volleyball.

There's no doubt you can strengthen and lift your buttocks. But just remember, if your rear end is squishier than you'd like, firming it up requires a two-pronged approach: tightening the muscles underneath and thinning out the layer of fat on top.

Muscle Basics

Your glutes are the three muscles that make up your buttocks and hips. The largest is the *gluteus maximus,* more commonly known as your buttocks. It's the muscle you use when you lift your leg behind you or rotate your thigh outward. The *gluteus medius* and *gluteus minimus* are located on the sides of your hips. It is these glute muscles that lift your leg out to the side; you don't actually have outer thigh muscles that do the job.

Week 3: The Plan

Workouts This Week: 2

Sets per Exercise: 1–2

Reps per Set: 12–15

Reps per Abdominal Set: 15–20

Toning Focus: Buttocks

TONING EXERCISE	PAGE
1. Hip Lift	220
2. Backward Lunge	222
3. Leg Lift	224
4. Seated Back Flye	236
5. Reverse Curl	212
6. Standing Side Lift	228
7. Push-up	238
8. Inner Thigh Pull	230
9. Rear Raise	246
10. Standing Calf Raise	256
11. Concentration Curl	254
12. French Press	248

Cardio Exercise
Calories to Burn: 450+
Total Days: 3+

Food Focus: Calories
Goal: Meet your Calorie Budget

TONING DAY 1

DATE _____

FOCUS: **Buttocks**

	SETS	REPS	WEIGHT
1. Hip Lift			
2. Backward Lunge			
3. Leg Lift			
4. Seated Back Flye			
5. Reverse Curl			
6. Standing Side Lift			
7. Push-up			
8. Inner Thigh Pull			
9. Rear Raise			
10. Standing Calf Raise			
11. Concentration Curl			
12. French Press			

TONING DAY 2

DATE _____

FOCUS: **Buttocks**

	SETS	REPS	WEIGHT
1. Hip Lift			
2. Backward Lunge			
3. Leg Lift			
4. Seated Back Flye			
5. Reverse Curl			
6. Standing Side Lift			
7. Push-up			
8. Inner Thigh Pull			
9. Rear Raise			
10. Standing Calf Raise			
11. Concentration Curl			
12. French Press			

TONING DAY 3

DATE _____

FOCUS: **Buttocks**

	SETS	REPS	WEIGHT
1. Hip Lift			
2. Backward Lunge			
3. Leg Lift			
4. Seated Back Flye			
5. Reverse Curl			
6. Standing Side Lift			
7. Push-up			
8. Inner Thigh Pull			
9. Rear Raise			
10. Standing Calf Raise			
11. Concentration Curl			
12. French Press			

Week 3 MONDAY   DATE

CARDIO EXERCISE   TIME   CALORIES BURNED

STRETCHING   YES   NO

NUTRITION   FAT BUDGET _____   CALORIE BUDGET _____

	FAT GRAMS	CALORIES
Breakfast:		
Snack:		
Lunch:		
Snack:		
Dinner:		
Notes: **Totals:**		

FOOD GROUP SERVINGS

Fruits ○ ○ ○ ○ ○
Vegetables ○ ○ ○ ○
Calcium-Rich ○ ○ ○
Protein-Rich ○ ○ ○ ○
Breads/Grains ○ ○ ○ ○ ○ ○ ○ ○ ○
Water ○ ○ ○ ○ ○ ○ ○ ○ ○

Food Fact

A great way to cut calories is to buy single-serving packages of snack foods. Or, if you buy the big, bargain-sized boxes, make your own single servings by scooping out smaller portions into plastic baggies.

Week 3 TUESDAY   DATE

CARDIO EXERCISE   TIME   CALORIES BURNED

STRETCHING YES   NO

NUTRITION FAT BUDGET _____ CALORIE BUDGET _____   FAT GRAMS   CALORIES

	FAT GRAMS	CALORIES
Breakfast:		
Snack:		
Lunch:		
Snack:		
Dinner:		
Notes: **Totals:**		

FOOD GROUP SERVINGS

Fruits ○ ○ ○ ○ ○
Vegetables ○ ○ ○ ○
Calcium-Rich ○ ○ ○
Protein-Rich ○ ○ ○ ○
Breads/Grains ○ ○ ○ ○ ○ ○ ○ ○ ○
Water ○ ○ ○ ○ ○ ○ ○ ○ ○

Food Fact

Spreading your calories throughout the day in small meals can help you stay alert. On the other hand, if you eat a huge lunch, you'll divert blood from your brain to your stomach to help with digestion. This will leave you feeling drowsy.

Week 3 WEDNESDAY DATE

CARDIO EXERCISE · TIME · CALORIES BURNED

STRETCHING YES [ ] NO [ ]

NUTRITION FAT BUDGET _____ CALORIE BUDGET _____

	FAT GRAMS	CALORIES
Breakfast:		
Snack:		
Lunch:		
Snack:		
Dinner:		
Notes: **Totals:**		

FOOD GROUP SERVINGS

Fruits ○○○○○
Vegetables ○○○○
Calcium-Rich ○○○
Protein-Rich ○○○○
Breads/Grains ○○○○○○○○○
Water ○○○○○○○○○

Fitness Tip

Don't focus on your body weight! A more meaningful number is your body fat percentage. For women, the optimal range is 18% to 26%; for men, 12% to 18%. Studies suggest that women who exceed 32% body fat, and men who exceed 22%, are at increased risk for heart disease, high blood pressure, and diabetes.

Week 3 THURSDAY   DATE _____

CARDIO EXERCISE   TIME   CALORIES BURNED

STRETCHING   YES ☐   NO ☐

NUTRITION   FAT BUDGET _____   CALORIE BUDGET _____

	FAT GRAMS	CALORIES
Breakfast:		
Snack:		
Lunch:		
Snack:		
Dinner:		
Notes: **Totals:**		

FOOD GROUP SERVINGS

Fruits   ○ ○ ○ ○ ○
Vegetables   ○ ○ ○ ○
Calcium-Rich   ○ ○ ○
Protein-Rich   ○ ○ ○ ○
Breads/Grains   ○ ○ ○ ○ ○ ○ ○ ○ ○
Water   ○ ○ ○ ○ ○ ○ ○ ○

Food Fact

A reminder that low-fat doesn't mean low-calorie: One Fat-Free Fig Newton has 50 calories, while a regular Fig Newton has 55 calories. One Reduced-Fat ChipsAhoy! cookie has 50 calories, while a regular ChipsAhoy! has 53 calories.

Week 3 FRIDAY

DATE [ ]

CARDIO EXERCISE

TIME

CALORIES BURNED

STRETCHING YES [ ]   No [ ]

NUTRITION FAT BUDGET _____   CALORIE BUDGET _____

	FAT GRAMS	CALORIES
Breakfast:		
Snack:		
Lunch:		
Snack:		
Dinner:		
Notes: Totals:		

FOOD GROUP SERVINGS

Fruits   ○ ○ ○ ○ ○
Vegetables   ○ ○ ○ ○
Calcium-Rich   ○ ○ ○
Protein-Rich   ○ ○ ○ ○
Breads/Grains   ○ ○ ○ ○ ○ ○ ○ ○ ○
Water   ○ ○ ○ ○ ○ ○ ○ ○

Fitness Tip

Be patient. You're not going to transform your body overnight. You'll notice strength gains within a few weeks, but it may take the entire 10 weeks (or beyond) to actually sculpt your muscles. Don't just focus on the results; enjoy the process.

Week 3 SATURDAY

DATE

CARDIO EXERCISE | TIME | CALORIES BURNED

STRETCHING YES [ ] No [ ]

NUTRITION FAT BUDGET _____ CALORIE BUDGET _____

	FAT GRAMS	CALORIES
Breakfast:		
Snack:		
Lunch:		
Snack:		
Dinner:		
Notes: **Totals:**		

FOOD GROUP SERVINGS

Fruits ○ ○ ○ ○ ○
Vegetables ○ ○ ○ ○
Calcium-Rich ○ ○ ○
Protein-Rich ○ ○ ○
Breads/Grains ○ ○ ○ ○ ○ ○ ○ ○
Water ○ ○ ○ ○ ○ ○ ○ ○

Food Fact

Bagels are growing! Calorie-counting books list the standard bagel at 2 ounces and 150 calories, but many new specialty bagels tip the scales at 4 to 5 ounces or more, boosting their calorie counts to between 300 and 550.

Week 3 SUNDAY   DATE [____]

CARDIO EXERCISE TIME CALORIES BURNED
[____] [____] [____]

STRETCHING YES [____] NO [____]

NUTRITION FAT BUDGET _____ CALORIE BUDGET _____

	FAT GRAMS	CALORIES
Breakfast:		
Snack:		
Lunch:		
Snack:		
Dinner:		
Notes: **Totals:**		

FOOD GROUP SERVINGS

Fruits ○ ○ ○ ○ ○
Vegetables ○ ○ ○ ○
Calcium-Rich ○ ○ ○
Protein-Rich ○ ○ ○ ○
Breads/Grains ○ ○ ○ ○ ○ ○ ○ ○ ○
Water ○ ○ ○ ○ ○ ○ ○ ○

Food Fact

Look closely at serving sizes when comparing food labels. Oreo cookies have 160 calories per serving, whereas Double Stuf Oreos have 140 calories. But the regular Oreo serving size is 3 cookies, while the Double Stuf serving size is just 2.

Week in Review

TONING

Days [ ] Did you meet the goal? _____

Notes _____

_____

CARDIO EXERCISE

Days [ ] Calories [ ] Did you meet the goals? _____

Notes _____

_____

WEIGHT [ ]

NUTRITION

Days Under Fat Budget [ ] Food Focus Rating, 1–5 [ ]

Remember that no matter what or how much is going on in your life, it will pass! Deal with the hectic demands of the moment, but don't let them dominate your life.

Kathy

CARBOHYDRATES
AND THIGHS

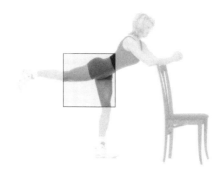

Carbohydrates

NUTRITION GOAL RECAP

This week, count your Quality Starch servings. Give yourself a point every time you choose a high-quality complex carbohydrate over a less nutritious one—for instance, wheat bread over white bread. I'm not giving you a numerical goal—just do your best!

grew up on white bread. My family used it for everything—cinnamon toast, ham sandwiches, French toast. It wasn't until college that I came to an important realization: this stuff isn't *food!* It has virtually no taste, and with that awful, pasty texture, it practically dissolves in your mouth. Nutritionally speaking, white bread is a zero. Whole wheat bread has 88 percent more fiber and magnesium, 62 percent more zinc, and 72 percent more chromium—to name just a few nutrients. Still, three out of every four loaves of bread sold in this country are white bread. It's not enough to replace high-fat foods with high-carbohydrate foods. The *quality* of your carbs is crucial. White bread and Pepsi are carbohydrates, but clearly, they're not going to keep you energized all day long, and they're not exactly loaded with nutrients. You need to distinguish the nutritious carbohydrates from the empty ones.

That's your goal for this week. Rather than count carbohydrate grams, you'll try extra hard to meet your fruit and vegetable serving recommendations. At the same time, you'll count your high-quality starch servings. In the Quality Starches column, give yourself a point for a half cup of brown rice, a slice of whole grain bread, or an ounce of Grape Nuts—but not for white rice, white bread, or Froot Loops. This will make you think carefully about your carb choices. (The white foods will still count when you fill in the circles for Starch servings at the bottom of the page.)

All carbohydrates have 4 calories per gram, compared to 9 calories per fat gram. But let's look more closely at the different types of carbs. You've probably heard about "complex" carbohydrates and "simple" ones. Complex carbs are starches in their natural forms—potatoes, rice, beans, pasta, whole wheat bread. Most complex carbohydrates are low in calories, low in fat, and high in fiber, and they make you feel full. The sugar in complex carbohydrates is absorbed slowly into your bloodstream, so your blood sugar level and energy level remain fairly constant.

On the other hand, simple carbohydrates—table sugar, honey, corn syrup—are absorbed quickly, causing the amount of sugar in your blood to skyrocket. In response, your pancreas pumps out more insulin to lower your blood sugar. But when your blood sugar shoots back down, often to a level below where you started, you feel tired and hungry. This is what nutritionists mean when they talk about sugar "highs" and "lows." Not only can refined, simple sugars wreak havoc with your blood sugar, but they also have no bulk to make you feel full. It's easy to just keep eating and eating and eating. Who ever got full on a Twinkie?

Now, not all foods containing simple sugars are bad for you. Most fruits, for instance, contain simple carbohydrates, and you'll never hear me steer you away from a banana. That's because these *natural, unrefined* simple sugars come packaged with vitamins, minerals, water, and fiber.

At the turn of the century, Americans got most of their carbs from complex sources such as grains and beans and natural simple sugars in fruits and vegetables. But today, we get more than half of our carbs from refined and processed sugars. This week, try to eat like your great-grandparents did!

Thighs

Think of someone you know who has lost weight simply by dieting. Now picture a friend who has included strength training in her weight-loss program. There's a big difference—and it's obvious when you look at their thighs. The diet-only person may have *thinner* legs than before, but the exerciser's thighs will have that terrific strength and tone.

My program targets your thighs from all four sides: the front, back, inside, and outside. Strong front thigh muscles are particularly helpful for preventing knee pain. Since your knees never really get a rest—they bend with every step—they're susceptible to aches and injury, especially with age. Strong quads help keep your kneecaps in line so you can walk, run, cycle, and climb without a second thought.

Meanwhile, toned rear thigh muscles give you that sexy sweep at the back of your legs. These muscles, along with your buttocks, are the real powerhouse of your lower body. They help push you forward when you walk and lift your body as you climb stairs. As for your inner and outer thighs, they don't get much of a workout unless you play tennis, skate, or do other activities that involve moving from side to side. It's important to take the time to target these muscles directly so they'll perform when you need them. If you were to slip on ice, for instance, strong inner thighs would contract to keep you upright, maybe even preventing a muscle pull.

If you're diligent about training all four sides of your thighs, the payoff will be tremendous. Everyone will know you've done a lot more than cut fat from your diet. They'll take one look at your thighs and know you've really been working out!

Muscle Basics

Your front thigh muscle group is the *quadriceps*. Your four quads are the *rectus femoris, vastus medialis, vastus lateralis,* and *vastus intermedius*. You have three *hamstrings,* or rear thigh muscles: *biceps femoris, semitendinosus,* and *semimembranosus*. You use your quads when you straighten your knees and your hamstrings when you bend them. As I mentioned in the buttocks chapter, you don't really have outer thigh muscles; it's your hip muscles that do the job of pulling your leg out to the side. The main muscles involved are the *gluteus medius, gluteus minimus,* and *tensor fasciae latae*. Together, they're referred to as your *abductors;* your inner thigh muscles are your *adductors*.

Week 4: The Plan

Workouts This Week: 2
Sets per Exercise: 1–2
Reps per Set: 12–15
Reps per Abdominal Set: 15–20
Toning Focus: Thighs

TONING EXERCISE	PAGE
1. Squat	226
2. Hamstring Curl	232
3. Inner Thigh Pull	230
4. Standing Side Lift	228
5. Seated Biceps Curl	252
6. Triceps Kickback	250
7. Crunch	210
8. Back Extension with a Twist	218
9. Chest Flye	240
10. Seated Back Flye	236
11. Lateral Raise	242
12. Standing Calf Raise	256

Cardio Exercise
Calories to Burn: 500+
Total Days: 3+

Food Focus: Carbohydrates
Goal: Count your Quality Starch servings

TONING DAY 1

DATE _____

FOCUS: **Thighs**

	SETS	REPS	WEIGHT
1. Squat			
2. Hamstring Curl			
3. Inner Thigh Pull			
4. Standing Side Lift			
5. Seated Biceps Curl			
6. Triceps Kickback			
7. Crunch			
8. Back Ext. with Twist			
9. Chest Flye			
10. Seated Back Flye			
11. Lateral Raise			
12. Standing Calf Raise			

TONING DAY 2

DATE _____

FOCUS: **Thighs**

	SETS	REPS	WEIGHT
1. Squat			
2. Hamstring Curl			
3. Inner Thigh Pull			
4. Standing Side Lift			
5. Seated Biceps Curl			
6. Triceps Kickback			
7. Crunch			
8. Back Ext. with Twist			
9. Chest Flye			
10. Seated Back Flye			
11. Lateral Raise			
12. Standing Calf Raise			

TONING DAY 3

DATE _____

FOCUS: **Thighs**

	SETS	REPS	WEIGHT
1. Squat			
2. Hamstring Curl			
3. Inner Thigh Pull			
4. Standing Side Lift			
5. Seated Biceps Curl			
6. Triceps Kickback			
7. Crunch			
8. Back Ext. with Twist			
9. Chest Flye			
10. Seated Back Flye			
11. Lateral Raise			
12. Standing Calf Raise			

Week 4 MONDAY   DATE

CARDIO EXERCISE   TIME   CALORIES BURNED

STRETCHING YES [ ]   NO [ ]

NUTRITION FAT BUDGET _____

	FAT GRAMS	QUALITY STARCHES
Breakfast:		
Snack:		
Lunch:		
Snack:		
Dinner:		
Notes: **Totals:**		

FOOD GROUP SERVINGS

Fruits   ○ ○ ○ ○ ○
Vegetables   ○ ○ ○ ○
Calcium-Rich   ○ ○ ○
Protein-Rich   ○ ○ ○ ○
Breads/Grains   ○ ○ ○ ○ ○ ○ ○ ○ ○
Water   ○ ○ ○ ○ ○ ○ ○ ○

Food Fact

Potatoes in their natural form are a nutritional bargain, full of vitamins and minerals. A half-pound baked potato has 170 calories, virtually none from fat; a quarter-pound of fries—a large at McDonald's—has 440 calories, 45 percent from fat!

Week 4 TUESDAY   DATE

CARDIO EXERCISE   TIME   CALORIES BURNED

STRETCHING YES ☐   NO ☐

NUTRITION FAT BUDGET _____

	FAT GRAMS	QUALITY STARCHES
Breakfast:		
Snack:		
Lunch:		
Snack:		
Dinner:		
Notes: **Totals:**		

FOOD GROUP SERVINGS

Fruits ○ ○ ○ ○ ○
Vegetables ○ ○ ○ ○
Calcium-Rich ○ ○ ○
Protein-Rich ○ ○ ○ ○
Breads/Grains ○ ○ ○ ○ ○ ○ ○ ○
Water ○ ○ ○ ○ ○ ○ ○ ○ ○

Food Fact

Eat carbohydrates within an hour of a long workout. If you wait longer to refuel, you won't recover as well for your next workout. If you're not hungry, drink your carbs in juice or fruit smoothies.

Week 4 WEDNESDAY DATE [ ]

CARDIO EXERCISE | TIME | CALORIES BURNED

[ ] | [ ] | [ ]

STRETCHING YES [ ] NO [ ]

NUTRITION FAT BUDGET _____

	FAT GRAMS	QUALITY STARCHES
Breakfast:		
Snack:		
Lunch:		
Snack:		
Dinner:		
Notes: **Totals:**		

FOOD GROUP SERVINGS

Fruits ○○○○○
Vegetables ○○○○
Calcium-Rich ○○○
Protein-Rich ○○○○
Breads/Grains ○○○○○○○○○
Water ○○○○○○○○○

Fitness Tip

Don't underestimate the benefits of short workouts. Sometimes I hear people say, "What's the point? I only have 15 minutes." Well, you can accomplish a lot in 15 minutes! Studies show that when it comes to health benefits, two 15-minute bouts of exercise are virtually as good as a full half hour.

Week 4 THURSDAY

DATE

CARDIO EXERCISE

TIME

CALORIES BURNED

STRETCHING YES   NO

NUTRITION FAT BUDGET _____

	FAT GRAMS	QUALITY STARCHES
Breakfast:		
Snack:		
Lunch:		
Snack:		
Dinner:		
Notes: **Totals:**		

FOOD GROUP SERVINGS

Fruits   ○ ○ ○ ○ ○
Vegetables   ○ ○ ○ ○
Calcium-Rich   ○ ○ ○
Protein-Rich   ○ ○ ○ ○
Breads/Grains   ○ ○ ○ ○ ○ ○ ○ ○ ○
Water   ○ ○ ○ ○ ○ ○ ○ ○ ○

Food Fact

We eat more fruit now than Americans did 100 years ago, but we eat one third less *fresh* fruit. Getting your fruit in Strawberry Newtons just isn't the same as eating a bowl of sliced fresh berries!

Week 4 FRIDAY

DATE

CARDIO EXERCISE

TIME

CALORIES BURNED

STRETCHING   YES ☐   NO ☐

NUTRITION   FAT BUDGET _____

	FAT GRAMS	QUALITY STARCHES
Breakfast:		
Snack:		
Lunch:		
Snack:		
Dinner:		
Notes: **Totals:**		

FOOD GROUP SERVINGS

Fruits   ○ ○ ○ ○ ○
Vegetables   ○ ○ ○ ○
Calcium-Rich   ○ ○ ○
Protein-Rich   ○ ○ ○ ○
Breads/Grains   ○ ○ ○ ○ ○ ○ ○ ○ ○
Water   ○ ○ ○ ○ ○ ○ ○ ○ ○

Fitness Tip

Your body keeps burning extra calories *after* your workouts. Experts aren't sure how long the "bonus" burn lasts—it may be less than an hour for aerobic workouts—but one thing is for sure: You won't get any bonus burn if you don't exercise!

Week 4 SATURDAY   DATE ☐

CARDIO EXERCISE   TIME   CALORIES BURNED

☐   ☐   ☐

STRETCHING YES ☐   NO ☐

NUTRITION FAT BUDGET _____

	FAT GRAMS	QUALITY STARCHES
Breakfast:		
Snack:		
Lunch:		
Snack:		
Dinner:		
Notes: **Totals:**		

FOOD GROUP SERVINGS

Fruits   ○ ○ ○ ○ ○
Vegetables   ○ ○ ○ ○
Calcium-Rich   ○ ○ ○
Protein-Rich   ○ ○ ○ ○
Breads/Grains   ○ ○ ○ ○ ○ ○ ○ ○ ○
Water   ○ ○ ○ ○ ○ ○ ○ ○

Food Fact

Foods with "enriched" flour are better than their nonenriched counterparts, but don't be fooled by the term. It means that some of the vitamins and minerals removed during processing have been added back, but the fiber hasn't. The real thing is always best.

Week 4 SUNDAY   DATE

CARDIO EXERCISE	TIME	CALORIES BURNED

STRETCHING   YES ☐   No ☐

NUTRITION   FAT BUDGET _____

	FAT GRAMS	QUALITY STARCHES
Breakfast:		
Snack:		
Lunch:		
Snack:		
Dinner:		
Notes: **Totals:**		

FOOD GROUP SERVINGS

Fruits   ○ ○ ○ ○ ○
Vegetables   ○ ○ ○ ○
Calcium-Rich   ○ ○ ○
Protein-Rich   ○ ○ ○ ○
Breads/Grains   ○ ○ ○ ○ ○ ○ ○ ○
Water   ○ ○ ○ ○ ○ ○ ○ ○

Food Fact

Be sure to buy bread labeled "100 percent whole wheat" or "whole grain." Other "wheat" or "grain" breads may actually contain mostly refined white flour that's been colored brown.

WEEK IN REVIEW

TONING

DAYS [   ]   DID YOU MEET THE GOAL? _____

NOTES _____

_____

CARDIO EXERCISE

DAYS [   ] CALORIES [   ]   DID YOU MEET THE GOALS? _____

NOTES _____

_____

WEIGHT [   ]

NUTRITION

DAYS UNDER FAT BUDGET [   ]   FOOD FOCUS RATING, 1–5 [   ]

Rigid, inflexible diets are recipes
for failure. My program isn't
a diet – it's a plan for sensible,
healthy eating. There's no need to
deprive yourself!
                        Kathy

PROTEIN
AND UPPER BACK

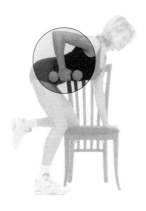

Protein

NUTRITION GOAL RECAP

This week, count your protein grams and aim to meet your Protein Goal—determined by multiplying your weight by .36. Remember: This isn't a maximum number; it's okay to go over.

Americans treat protein two different ways: On the one hand, most people get far more than they need—and from sources, like steak and cheese, that are loaded with fat. On the other hand, I've noticed a segment of obsessive dieters who equate protein with fat, so they eat none at all! Well, there's a simple solution for everyone: low-fat, high-protein foods. With all the low-fat dairy products and extra-lean meats available, it's easy to get your protein without all the fat. A half cup of low-fat cottage cheese has the same amount of protein as a 2.5-ounce hamburger; but the burger has nearly three times the fat and 50 percent more calories!

Protein is vital because it's made up of amino acids, which your body uses to build and repair your muscles, tendons, red blood cells, and enzymes. Your body needs more than twenty different amino acids, eleven of which it can produce on its own. However, the remaining nine must come from the food you eat. These are called "essential" amino acids.

How much protein do you really need? The Recommended Dietary Allowance for protein is .36 grams per 1 pound of body weight. To figure out my protein needs, I multiply my weight—130 pounds—by .36. I need about 47 grams. This week you'll count protein grams to see how you stack up. But, remember, unlike your Fat Budget, your Protein Goal is not a maximum number; it's okay to get more (but not *too* much more). All food labels include protein information; however, it'll be tougher to count grams in nonpackaged foods because most fat-gram books don't include protein information. To fill in the gaps, you can use the following chart to approximate your protein values:

AVERAGE PROTEIN CONTENT OF FOODS

SOURCE	AMOUNT	PROTEIN GRAMS
Legumes, cooked	1 cup	12 grams
Milk, yogurt	1 cup	8–10 grams
Meat, fish, poultry, cheese	1 ounce	7 grams
Most starches	1/2 cup	3 grams
Vegetables	1/2 cup	2 grams

But watch out for the fat that may come along with your protein. Some animal sources of protein actually contain more fat calories than protein calories; 4 ounces of lean ground beef (83 percent lean) is 39 percent protein and *61 percent* fat! Most vegetable sources, on the other hand, come packed with complex carbohydrates. Experts say we should get two-thirds of our protein from plant sources and one-third from animal sources; yet most of us do just the opposite. The richest sources of vegetable protein are legumes—dried peas and beans, including lentils, blackeyed peas, soybeans, kidney beans, pinto beans, and black beans.

One caution, however: If you are a vegetarian or get most of your protein from plant sources, you must choose your protein sources carefully. Meat, chicken, fish, eggs, and milk products contain all of the essential amino acids, but the protein in most plant sources is "incomplete," meaning it's missing one or another amino acid. You can easily rectify this situation by combining two incomplete proteins that complement each other. You don't need to eat "complementary" proteins in the same meal, just a variety of different protein sources on a regular basis. Here are some combinations that'll do the trick:

COMPLEMENTARY PROTEINS

Rice with: cheese, beans, or sesame

Wheat with: beans, peanuts and milk, or soybean

Corn with: beans

Beans with: wheat or corn

If you find that you're getting a lot more protein than you need, try what my family has done: Rearrange your meals. Dinner doesn't need to revolve around a big hunk of meat or large portions of chicken. We use small strips of chicken on our pasta primavera and sprinkle extra-lean turkey meat in our spaghetti sauce. Believe me, a little meat, fish, or chicken can go a long way.

Upper Back

When you think about reshaping your body, you probably focus on slimming this area or tightening that one. But you can change your appearance by *building,* too! The upper back is a great example. By developing these large muscles on top, you can make your waist, hips, and lower back seem smaller.

Until a few years ago, I didn't pay much attention to my upper back muscles. That sure changed after my daughter Perrie was born. Suddenly, my business was busier than ever, I was doing frequent TV appearances—and I was always carrying around a 25-pound child! Meanwhile, I noticed a constant soreness in my upper back and neck area. It was stress. If your upper back muscles aren't strong, they'll bear the brunt of your tension. Now I'm devoted to my back exercises. I'm always adding new moves to my routine, and I don't feel the strain when my life gets busy.

Powerful upper back muscles will also help out if you're a desk jockey. Sitting all day long can take a toll on your posture, a problem that's exacerbated when your upper back muscles are weak. If you strengthen them, you'll counteract that tendency to slouch. You'll stand tall and project a strong image.

Muscle Basics

Your largest back muscle is your *latissimus dorsi.* You use your lats when you pull a heavy box down from a high shelf or when you pull apart two grocery carts that are stuck together. Above your lats are your traps—officially known as your *trapezius.* When you lift a heavy suitcase, your trapezius bears a lot of the weight so you don't strain your shoulders. Your *rhomboids* pull your shoulder blades together and help you maintain perfect posture.

Week 5: The Plan

Workouts This Week: 2
Sets per Exercise: 2
Reps per Set: 12–15
Reps per Abdominal Set: 15–20
Toning Focus: Upper Back

TONING EXERCISE	PAGE
1. One-Arm Row	234
2. Seated Back Flye	236
3. Push-up	238
4. Leg Lift	224
5. Squat	226
6. Front Raise	244
7. French Press	248
8. Cross Crunch	214
9. Back Extension with a Twist	218
10. Standing Side Lift	228
11. Inner Thigh Pull	230
12. Toe Raise	258

Cardio Exercise
Calories to Burn: 550+
Total Days: 3+

Food Focus: Protein
Goal: Count your protein grams and meet your Protein Goal

TONING DAY 1

DATE _____

FOCUS: **Upper Back**

	SETS	REPS	WEIGHT
1. One-Arm Row			
2. Seated Back Flye			
3. Push-up			
4. Leg Lift			
5. Squat			
6. Front Raise			
7. French Press			
8. Cross Crunch			
9. Back Ext. with Twist			
10. Standing Side Lift			
11. Inner Thigh Pull			
12. Toe Raise			

TONING DAY 2

DATE _____

FOCUS: **Upper Back**

	SETS	REPS	WEIGHT
1. One-Arm Row			
2. Seated Back Flye			
3. Push-up			
4. Leg Lift			
5. Squat			
6. Front Raise			
7. French Press			
8. Cross Crunch			
9. Back Ext. with Twist			
10. Standing Side Lift			
11. Inner Thigh Pull			
12. Toe Raise			

TONING DAY 3

DATE _____

FOCUS: **Upper Back**

	SETS	REPS	WEIGHT
1. One-Arm Row			
2. Seated Back Flye			
3. Push-up			
4. Leg Lift			
5. Squat			
6. Front Raise			
7. French Press			
8. Cross Crunch			
9. Back Ext. with Twist			
10. Standing Side Lift			
11. Inner Thigh Pull			
12. Toe Raise			

Week 5 MONDAY

DATE

CARDIO EXERCISE

TIME

CALORIES BURNED

STRETCHING YES ___ NO ___

NUTRITION FAT BUDGET _____ PROTEIN GOAL _____

	FAT GRAMS	PROTEIN GRAMS
Breakfast:		
Snack:		
Lunch:		
Snack:		
Dinner:		
Notes: **Totals:**		

FOOD GROUP SERVINGS

Fruits ○ ○ ○ ○ ○
Vegetables ○ ○ ○ ○
Calcium-Rich ○ ○ ○
Protein-Rich ○ ○ ○ ○
Breads/Grains ○ ○ ○ ○ ○ ○ ○ ○ ○
Water ○ ○ ○ ○ ○ ○ ○ ○

Food Fact

If all your meals include a mix of carbohydrates and protein, you'll stay satisfied a lot longer than if you eat carbohydrates alone. Eating protein an hour or so before a workout can help you stay energized!

Week 5 TUESDAY   DATE

CARDIO EXERCISE   TIME   CALORIES BURNED

STRETCHING   YES   NO

NUTRITION   FAT BUDGET _____   PROTEIN GOAL _____

	FAT GRAMS	PROTEIN GRAMS
Breakfast:		
Snack:		
Lunch:		
Snack:		
Dinner:		
Notes: **Totals:**		

FOOD GROUP SERVINGS

Fruits	○ ○ ○ ○ ○
Vegetables	○ ○ ○ ○
Calcium-Rich	○ ○ ○
Protein-Rich	○ ○ ○ ○
Breads/Grains	○ ○ ○ ○ ○ ○ ○ ○ ○
Water	○ ○ ○ ○ ○ ○ ○ ○

Food Fact

If you severely restrict your calorie intake, you begin to break down muscle for energy. Because your body is constantly turning over protein and doesn't store it, you need to restock every day.

Week 5 WEDNESDAY DATE

CARDIO EXERCISE   TIME   CALORIES BURNED

STRETCHING YES [ ] NO [ ]

NUTRITION FAT BUDGET _____ PROTEIN GOAL _____

	FAT GRAMS	PROTEIN GRAMS
Breakfast:		
Snack:		
Lunch:		
Snack:		
Dinner:		
Notes: **Totals:**		

FOOD GROUP SERVINGS

Fruits ○ ○ ○ ○ ○
Vegetables ○ ○ ○ ○
Calcium-Rich ○ ○ ○
Protein-Rich ○ ○ ○ ○
Breads/Grains ○ ○ ○ ○ ○ ○ ○ ○ ○
Water ○ ○ ○ ○ ○ ○ ○ ○

Fitness Tip

If you keep doing the same toning routine in the same order, not only will you get bored—so will your muscles! If you let your muscles adapt to a certain program, they'll no longer be stimulated to keep getting stronger.

Week 5 THURSDAY   DATE

CARDIO EXERCISE   TIME   CALORIES BURNED

STRETCHING   YES   NO

NUTRITION   FAT BUDGET _____   PROTEIN GOAL _____

	FAT GRAMS	PROTEIN GRAMS
Breakfast:		
Snack:		
Lunch:		
Snack:		
Dinner:		
Notes: **Totals:**		

FOOD GROUP SERVINGS

Fruits   ○ ○ ○ ○ ○
Vegetables   ○ ○ ○ ○
Calcium-Rich   ○ ○ ○
Protein-Rich   ○ ○ ○ ○
Breads/Grains   ○ ○ ○ ○ ○ ○ ○ ○ ○
Water   ○ ○ ○ ○ ○ ○ ○ ○

Food Fact

Many people don't get enough protein in the morning. Try adding an egg, lean ham, low-fat cheese, or low-fat cottage cheese to your breakfast, and you'll feel satisfied longer.

Week 5 FRIDAY   DATE [ ]

CARDIO EXERCISE   TIME   CALORIES BURNED

[ ]   [ ]   [ ]

STRETCHING YES [ ]   NO [ ]

NUTRITION FAT BUDGET _____ PROTEIN GOAL _____

	FAT GRAMS	PROTEIN GRAMS
Breakfast:		
Snack:		
Lunch:		
Snack:		
Dinner:		
Notes: **Totals:**		

FOOD GROUP SERVINGS

Fruits   ○ ○ ○ ○ ○
Vegetables   ○ ○ ○ ○
Calcium-Rich   ○ ○ ○
Protein-Rich   ○ ○ ○ ○
Breads/Grains   ○ ○ ○ ○ ○ ○ ○ ○ ○
Water   ○ ○ ○ ○ ○ ○ ○ ○

Fitness Tip

On days when you don't do any toning or aerobic exercise, take a five-minute walk and follow it with five minutes of stretching. You'll be amazed at how much better you feel with so little time and effort. You'll also have something to write in your log!

Week 5 SATURDAY DATE

CARDIO EXERCISE   TIME   CALORIES BURNED

STRETCHING   YES   NO

NUTRITION FAT BUDGET _____ PROTEIN GOAL _____

	FAT GRAMS	PROTEIN GRAMS
Breakfast:		
Snack:		
Lunch:		
Snack:		
Dinner:		
Notes: **Totals:**		

FOOD GROUP SERVINGS

Fruits	○ ○ ○ ○ ○
Vegetables	○ ○ ○ ○
Calcium-Rich	○ ○ ○
Protein-Rich	○ ○ ○ ○
Breads/Grains	○ ○ ○ ○ ○ ○ ○ ○ ○
Water	○ ○ ○ ○ ○ ○ ○ ○

Food Fact

Serious athletes may need more protein than the average person. But you can easily get enough from your food without using protein powders, pills, or other products. Most people consume 150 percent to 200 percent of the RDA for protein in their food alone.

Week 5 SUNDAY DATE

CARDIO EXERCISE TIME CALORIES BURNED

STRETCHING YES NO

NUTRITION FAT BUDGET _____ PROTEIN GOAL _____

	FAT GRAMS	PROTEIN GRAMS
Breakfast:		
Snack:		
Lunch:		
Snack:		
Dinner:		
Notes: **Totals:**		

FOOD GROUP SERVINGS

Fruits ○ ○ ○ ○ ○
Vegetables ○ ○ ○ ○
Calcium-Rich ○ ○ ○
Protein-Rich ○ ○ ○ ○
Breads/Grains ○ ○ ○ ○ ○ ○ ○ ○ ○ ○
Water ○ ○ ○ ○ ○ ○ ○ ○ ○

Food Fact

The big myth about vegetarian diets is that they don't supply enough protein. Most vegetarian menus contain plenty of protein from dairy products, eggs, grains, beans, and nuts as long as total calorie intake is adequate and the proteins balanced. Vegans—vegetarians who don't eat dairy products—also can get adequate protein, but they need to plan their diet more carefully.

WEEK IN REVIEW

TONING

DAYS [　　　]　　　DID YOU MEET THE GOAL? _____

NOTES _____

_____

CARDIO EXERCISE

DAYS [　　　] CALORIES [　　　] DID YOU MEET THE GOALS? _____

NOTES _____

_____

WEIGHT [　　　]

NUTRITION

DAYS UNDER FAT BUDGET [　　　]　　FOOD FOCUS RATING, 1–5 [　　　]

you've made it halfway through your log. Now reward yourself — with a new scarf, fresh flowers for the house, or an entire day all to yourself. you've earned it!

Kathy

C ALCIUM
AND C HEST

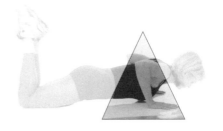

Calcium

Growing up, we all heard our parents say, "Drink your milk so you'll have strong bones!" But I don't think any of us, our parents included, realized just how important that advice was. In fact, only in recent years have scientists focused on the devastating effects of bone loss—and the important role that calcium can play in preventing it.

First, a few facts that stunned me:

• Roughly 25 million Americans have osteoporosis, a disease of accelerated bone loss. Four out of five are women.

• Osteoporosis causes 1.5 million fractures a year, mostly of the back, hip, and wrist. When a bone is extremely weak, it doesn't even take a fall to fracture it. Bending over to pick up a baby could be enough.

• Fifteen percent of white women age 50 or older will fracture a hip sometime in their life. (African-American women suffer fewer fractures because they have genetically denser bones.) Among those age 75 or older, as many as 20 percent will die within a year after the fracture. Only one out of five fully recover.

But none of this is inevitable! On the contrary, osteoporosis is highly preventable. Studies show you can ward off the disease by taking a three-pronged approach: 1) lifting weights regularly, 2) doing "weight-bearing" exercise (activities, such as walking and aerobics, in which your feet touch the ground), and 3) consuming sufficient calcium.

This week your nutrition goal is to get at least 800 milligrams of calcium a day. You can generally achieve this by eating three servings of dairy products, but calcium comes from other sources, too. I think it's instructive to spend a week actually counting your calcium milligrams to see if you're making the grade. Studies show that most women get only half the calcium they need. In addition to reading food labels this week, use the following chart to estimate your calcium intake.

CALCIUM INTAKE

CALCIUM FOOD SOURCES	CALCIUM (IN MILLIGRAMS)
Plain, nonfat yogurt (1 cup)	500
Skim milk (1 cup)	352
Calcium-enriched orange juice (1 cup)	300
Swiss cheese (1 ounce)	272
Cheddar cheese (1 ounce)	204
Ice cream or ice milk (1 cup)	164
Tofu (3 ounces)	150
Soybeans (1/2 cup cooked)	88
Low-fat (2 percent) cottage cheese (1/2 cup)	77
Grated Parmesan cheese (1 tablespoon)	69
Orange (1 medium)	52
Whole wheat or white bread (2 slices)	47
Pinto beans (1/2 cup cooked)	41
Broccoli (1/2 cup cooked, chopped)	36
Sweet potato (1 medium baked)	32

So what exactly will calcium do to your bones? Well, that depends on how old you are. When you're young, calcium will help you *build* bone. But by age 35, you've developed as much bone as you're ever going to have. (In fact, by age 18, you've already reached 95 percent of your maximum bone density.) After age 35, your goal is to *maintain* as much of your bone mass as possible. If you don't exercise and get enough calcium, you'll lose one-half to 1 percent of bone mass each year until menopause; after that, a woman's rate of bone loss tends to double for five years before leveling off. But the good news is, if you do everything right, you can slow your rate of bone loss significantly—by about 50 percent, maybe even more. Ultimately, your goal is to have banked away enough bone so that when the inevitable bone loss kicks in, you'll have plenty left over.

Chest

You might not realize this, but chest exercises can do wonders for your bustline. They're not going to change the size or shape of your breasts, but since your chest muscles help support your breasts, you can definitely give your chest a lift! Looks aside, a strong chest will give you a little extra oomph when you wash your car, mow the lawn, or push an overloaded shopping cart.

My favorite chest exercise is the push-up. I used to think push-ups were for men only; after all, no one expects women to be strong enough to do them. Most men have more upper body strength than women, but I've built enough chest strength to do 3 sets of 12 full-fledged push-ups. That's more than some men I know!

Of course, it didn't happen overnight. When I decided to focus on strengthening my chest, I naturally started out doing push-ups on my knees. After a few months, I decided to try one push-up on my toes, and much to my surprise, I could do it! From that point on, I'd start each set with a couple of full push-ups, then finish with 10 or 12 reps in the modified stance. Soon I was doing half and half, and eventually I was doing them all on my toes. You just might be amazed at the potential strength hiding in your chest!

Muscle Basics

Your largest chest muscle is your *pectoralis major;* underneath are the *pectoralis minor* and the *serratus anterior*. You use your pecs whenever you push or carry something. Strong pecs also come in handy when you have to support your body weight, such as when you're on your hands and knees wiping up a spill on the kitchen floor.

Week 6: The Plan

Workouts This Week: 2

Sets per Exercise: 2

Reps per Set: 12–15

Reps per Abdominal Set: 15–20

Toning Focus: Chest

TONING EXERCISE	PAGE
1. Push-up	238
2. Chest Flye	240
3. One-Arm Row	234
4. Backward Lunge	222
5. Hamstring Curl	232
6. Reverse Curl	212
7. Back Extension	216
8. Seated Biceps Curl	252
9. Rear Raise	246
10. Hip Lift	220
11. Lateral Raise	242
12. Standing Calf Raise	256

Cardio Exercise

Calories to Burn: 600+

Total Days: 3–4+

Food Focus: Calcium

Goal: At least 800 milligrams of calcium a day

TONING DAY 1

DATE _____

FOCUS: **Chest**

	SETS	REPS	WEIGHT
1. Push-up			
2. Chest Flye			
3. One-Arm Row			
4. Backward Lunge			
5. Hamstring Curl			
6. Reverse Curl			
7. Back Extension			
8. Seated Biceps Curl			
9. Rear Raise			
10. Hip Lift			
11. Lateral Raise			
12. Standing Calf Raise			

TONING DAY 2

DATE _____

FOCUS: **Chest**

	SETS	REPS	WEIGHT
1. Push-up			
2. Chest Flye			
3. One-Arm Row			
4. Backward Lunge			
5. Hamstring Curl			
6. Reverse Curl			
7. Back Extension			
8. Seated Biceps Curl			
9. Rear Raise			
10. Hip Lift			
11. Lateral Raise			
12. Standing Calf Raise			

TONING DAY 3

Date _____

Focus: **Chest**

	SETS	REPS	WEIGHT
1. Push-up			
2. Chest Flye			
3. One-Arm Row			
4. Backward Lunge			
5. Hamstring Curl			
6. Reverse Curl			
7. Back Extension			
8. Seated Biceps Curl			
9. Rear Raise			
10. Hip Lift			
11. Lateral Raise			
12. Standing Calf Raise			

Week 6 MONDAY   DATE [ ]

CARDIO EXERCISE   TIME   CALORIES BURNED
[ ]   [ ]   [ ]

STRETCHING YES [ ]   NO [ ]

NUTRITION FAT BUDGET _____ CALCIUM _____

	FAT GRAMS	CALCIUM MG
Breakfast:		
Snack:		
Lunch:		
Snack:		
Dinner:		
Notes: **Totals:**		

FOOD GROUP SERVINGS

Fruits ○○○○○
Vegetables ○○○○
Calcium-Rich ○○○
Protein-Rich ○○○○
Breads/Grains ○○○○○○○○○
Water ○○○○○○○○

Food Fact

Researchers disagree about exactly how much calcium you need. The Recommended Dietary Allowance for people ages 25 to 55 is 800 milligrams a day. The Osteoporosis Foundation recommends 1,000 milligrams a day—and 1,500 milligrams for women over 55.

Week 6 TUESDAY   DATE [ ]

CARDIO EXERCISE   TIME   CALORIES BURNED
[ ]   [ ]   [ ]

STRETCHING   YES [ ]   NO [ ]

NUTRITION   FAT BUDGET _____   CALCIUM _____

	FAT GRAMS	CALCIUM MG
Breakfast:		
Snack:		
Lunch:		
Snack:		
Dinner:		
Notes: **Totals:**		

FOOD GROUP SERVINGS

Fruits	○ ○ ○ ○ ○
Vegetables	○ ○ ○ ○
Calcium-Rich	○ ○ ○
Protein-Rich	○ ○ ○
Breads/Grains	○ ○ ○ ○ ○ ○ ○ ○ ○
Water	○ ○ ○ ○ ○ ○ ○ ○

Food Fact
Osteoporosis costs the United States $10–$12 billion a year in related medical costs. Because our population is aging, this figure is expected to hit $60–$80 billion by 2025.

Week 6 WEDNESDAY DATE _____

CARDIO EXERCISE

	TIME	CALORIES BURNED

STRETCHING YES ☐ NO ☐

NUTRITION FAT BUDGET _____ CALCIUM _____

	FAT GRAMS	CALCIUM MG
Breakfast:		
Snack:		
Lunch:		
Snack:		
Dinner:		
Notes: **Totals:**		

FOOD GROUP SERVINGS

Fruits ○ ○ ○ ○ ○
Vegetables ○ ○ ○ ○
Calcium-Rich ○ ○ ○
Protein-Rich ○ ○ ○ ○
Breads/Grains ○ ○ ○ ○ ○ ○ ○ ○ ○
Water ○ ○ ○ ○ ○ ○ ○ ○

Fitness Tip

At some point during the program, you'll probably need to graduate to heavier dumbbells. Don't be afraid to do this—your muscles won't get bulky! However, just make sure you increase the amount of weight slowly.

Week 6 THURSDAY   DATE [ ]

CARDIO EXERCISE   TIME   CALORIES BURNED
[ ] [ ] [ ]

STRETCHING   YES [ ]   NO [ ]

NUTRITION   FAT BUDGET _____   CALCIUM _____

	FAT GRAMS	CALCIUM MG
Breakfast:		
Snack:		
Lunch:		
Snack:		
Dinner:		
Notes: **Totals:**		

FOOD GROUP SERVINGS

Fruits   ○ ○ ○ ○ ○
Vegetables   ○ ○ ○ ○
Calcium-Rich   ○ ○ ○
Protein-Rich   ○ ○ ○ ○
Breads/Grains   ○ ○ ○ ○ ○ ○ ○ ○ ○
Water   ○ ○ ○ ○ ○ ○ ○ ○

Food Fact

Look for a calcium supplement that mentions osteoporosis on the label. The Food and Drug Administration won't allow manufacturers to make claims about osteoporosis unless the tablet meets certain standards. Avoid "natural-source" calcium pills, such as oyster shell and bone meal, because they may contain lead.

Week 6 FRIDAY   DATE

CARDIO EXERCISE   TIME   CALORIES BURNED

STRETCHING YES   NO

NUTRITION FAT BUDGET _____   CALCIUM _____

	FAT GRAMS	CALCIUM MG
Breakfast:		
Snack:		
Lunch:		
Snack:		
Dinner:		
Notes: **Totals:**		

FOOD GROUP SERVINGS

Fruits   ○ ○ ○ ○ ○
Vegetables   ○ ○ ○ ○
Calcium-Rich   ○ ○ ○
Protein-Rich   ○ ○ ○ ○
Breads/Grains   ○ ○ ○ ○ ○ ○ ○ ○ ○
Water   ○ ○ ○ ○ ○ ○ ○ ○

Fitness Tip

How far you can move a joint largely depends on how tight your muscles are. Your knee, for instance, can move only as far as your calf and thigh muscles will allow. By making stretching a habit, you can keep your body loose and flexible for decades to come. This is key—as we age, our tissues tend to lose elasticity.

Week 6 SATURDAY   DATE [　　　]

CARDIO EXERCISE   TIME   CALORIES BURNED
[　　　]   [　　　]   [　　　]

STRETCHING YES [　]   NO [　]

NUTRITION FAT BUDGET _____ CALCIUM _____

	FAT GRAMS	CALCIUM MG
Breakfast:		
Snack:		
Lunch:		
Snack:		
Dinner:		
Notes: **Totals:**		

FOOD GROUP SERVINGS

Fruits   ○ ○ ○ ○ ○
Vegetables   ○ ○ ○ ○
Calcium-Rich   ○ ○ ○
Protein-Rich   ○ ○ ○ ○
Breads/Grains   ○ ○ ○ ○ ○ ○ ○ ○ ○
Water   ○ ○ ○ ○ ○ ○ ○ ○

Food Fact

White, fair-skinned, small-boned women have the greatest risk of osteoporosis. Men get osteoporosis less often than women do because their bones are dense and because they die younger. However, as more men live longer, the disease probably will become more of a problem for them.

Week 6   SUNDAY   DATE

CARDIO EXERCISE   TIME   CALORIES BURNED

STRETCHING   YES   NO

NUTRITION   FAT BUDGET _____   CALCIUM _____

	FAT GRAMS	CALCIUM MG
Breakfast:		
Snack:		
Lunch:		
Snack:		
Dinner:		
Notes: **Totals:**		

FOOD GROUP SERVINGS

Fruits   ○ ○ ○ ○ ○
Vegetables   ○ ○ ○ ○
Calcium-Rich   ○ ○ ○
Protein-Rich   ○ ○ ○
Breads/Grains   ○ ○ ○ ○ ○ ○ ○ ○
Water   ○ ○ ○ ○ ○ ○ ○ ○

Food Fact

Milk, cheese, and yogurt are by far the best sources of calcium in the typical American diet. Your body can absorb far more calcium from dairy products than from other food sources. For instance, only 5 percent of the calcium in spinach is absorbed, compared to 40 percent of the calcium in milk.

Week in Review

TONING

Days ☐   Did you meet the goal? _____

Notes _____

_____

CARDIO EXERCISE

Days ☐   Calories ☐   Did you meet the goals? _____

Notes _____

_____

WEIGHT ☐

NUTRITION

Days Under Fat Budget ☐   Food Focus Rating, 1–5

> I constantly hear people say, "I wish I'd worked out today." But I never hear anyone say, "I wish I hadn't worked out." Keep in mind that you'll always feel better in the end.
>
> *Kathy*

F I B E R
A N D   S H O U L D E R S

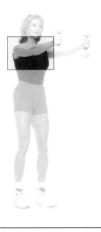

Fiber

NUTRITION GOAL RECAP

This week, your goal is to get at least 25 grams of fiber a day. This may take extra effort—the average American gets only 10 to 15.

love to feel full. I'm not talking about being stuffed—I enjoy that soothing, *satisfied* feeling that comes from eating just enough food. If I don't eat to the point of fullness, well, I just feel kind of edgy and distracted. To me, the best way to achieve this sense of contentment is to load up on high-fiber foods, such as grains, fruits, and vegetables. They're bulky *and* low in fat, so you can feel full without compromising your weight. As you probably know, fiber also helps keep you regular. And now research is pointing to two other reasons to make high-fiber foods a staple of your diet: They help prevent heart disease and colon cancer.

But first, what exactly *is* fiber? Actually, it's a term that covers a whole group of compounds that your body does not digest. Fiber comes only from plant foods, not animal products, and most of us don't get nearly enough of it to make a difference in our health. Experts recommend at least 25 grams of fiber a day, but the typical American gets only 10 to 15 grams. Your goal this week is to hit the 25 mark, and you're free to go over!

Don't worry—this doesn't mean you have to live on wheat bran for a week. When most of us think of fiber, it's the brown stuff that first comes to mind—foods like wheat bran, oat bran, barley, pinto beans, and lentils. But fiber comes in many colors and textures. Apples, blueberries, and apricots are good sources of fiber, whereas some of those crunchy brown foods are deceiving. You get only one-half gram of fiber from seven Nabisco Harvest Crisps 5-Grain crackers; a Snickers candy bar has twice the fiber! But that doesn't make the Snickers bar a good choice. The candy bar has nearly as much fiber as, say, a half a peach—but it has seven times the calories, not to mention plenty of fat.

The best way to get your fiber is through *unprocessed* high-fiber foods. Not only are these choices low in fat, but they're packed with vitamins and minerals. Researchers suspect that it might not be fiber alone that lowers the risk of heart disease and cancer, but rather the interaction of fiber with other components in these foods, such as vitamin C or E. In other words, choose a cup of strawberries over the strawberry-flavored Fi-Bar.

This week, in addition to reading labels on your cereal boxes, bread loaves, and soup cans, use the following fruit and vegetable charts to estimate your fiber intake.

FIBER INTAKE

FRUIT	FIBER GRAMS
Apple or pear	4
Apricots, dried, 1/3 cup	4
Blueberries, 1 cup	4
Banana or orange	3
Strawberries, 1 cup	3
Grapefruit, 1/2	2
Nectarine or peach	2

VEGETABLES AND LEGUMES (SERVING SIZE: 1/2 CUP)	
Beans	5–8
Lentils	7
Green peas	4
Baked or sweet potato with skin	4
Carrots	3
Asparagus or broccoli	2
Spinach or cabbage	2
Cauliflower or green beans	2
Celery or green pepper	1

Aim to eat a wide variety of high-fiber foods because the two categories of fiber—soluble and insoluble—have different functions and benefits, and no single food will give you all the fiber you need for good health. Soluble fibers, such as those found in fruit, oat bran, and cooked beans, may reduce your risk for heart disease by lowering your blood cholesterol. Insoluble fibers—found in wheat bran, whole grains, and vegetables—are the ones that reduce constipation. They hold on to water and speed the movement of waste products through your digestive tract. Research suggests that they may also reduce your risk of colon cancer. So this week—and in the weeks to come—get your fill of fiber!

Shoulders

When you start a strength-training program, one of the first places you'll see definition is in your shoulders. That's because most of us store relatively little fat in this area. Your newly toned shoulder muscles won't be hiding. You'll be so thrilled with your results that you just might go out and reward yourself with a new sleeveless dress!

Building up your shoulders, like firming your upper back muscles, can help make your body look more in proportion if you are larger on the bottom than on top. Well-developed shoulders will make you appear taller, and give you a real sense of presence. You'll also notice how nicely your clothes drape over your shoulders. I'm lucky that I have naturally broad shoulders—when shoulder pads were popular, I never had to wear them! Nevertheless, I've put in plenty of time toning and shaping this part of my body.

Although the front portion of your shoulders is naturally most noticeable, don't forget to work on the rear and the sides, which tend to be weaker. That's because they get less of a workout in daily life. You raise your arms forward a lot more often than you bring them back or out to the side. Strong rear shoulder muscles can help correct a slumping posture. If they're toned, they'll do their share of the work in keeping your shoulder blades back and down.

Muscle Basics

Your shoulder muscle—the *deltoid*—has three heads. The front (anterior) head helps raise your arm forward, while your rear (posterior) delt performs the reverse motion. Your middle (medial) deltoid lifts your arm to the side and helps the other two heads in their movements.

Week 7: The Plan

Workouts This Week: 2
Sets per Exercise: 2
Reps per Set: 12–15
Reps per Abdominal Set: 15–20
Toning Focus: Shoulders

TONING EXERCISE	PAGE
1. Front Raise	244
2. Lateral Raise	242
3. Rear Raise	246
4. Chest Flye	240
5. Concentration Curl	254
6. Triceps Kickback	250
7. Crunch	210
8. Back Extension with a Twist	218
9. Leg Lift	224
10. Squat	226
11. Inner Thigh Pull	230
12. Standing Side Lift	228

Cardio Exercise
Calories to Burn: 650+
Total Days: 3–4+

Food Focus: Fiber
Goal: At least 25 grams of fiber a day

TONING DAY 1

DATE _____

Focus: **Shoulders**

	SETS	REPS	WEIGHT
1. Front Raise			
2. Lateral Raise			
3. Rear Raise			
4. Chest Flye			
5. Concentration Curl			
6. Triceps Kickback			
7. Crunch			
8. Back Ext. with Twist			
9. Leg Lift			
10. Squat			
11. Inner Thigh Pull			
12. Standing Side Lift			

TONING DAY 2

DATE _____

FOCUS: **Shoulders**

	SETS	REPS	WEIGHT
1. Front Raise			
2. Lateral Raise			
3. Rear Raise			
4. Chest Flye			
5. Concentration Curl			
6. Triceps Kickback			
7. Crunch			
8. Back Ext. with Twist			
9. Leg Lift			
10. Squat			
11. Inner Thigh Pull			
12. Standing Side Lift			

TONING DAY 3

DATE _____

FOCUS: **Shoulders**

	SETS	REPS	WEIGHT
1. Front Raise			
2. Lateral Raise			
3. Rear Raise			
4. Chest Flye			
5. Concentration Curl			
6. Triceps Kickback			
7. Crunch			
8. Back Ext. with Twist			
9. Leg Lift			
10. Squat			
11. Inner Thigh Pull			
12. Standing Side Lift			

Week 7 MONDAY

DATE _____

CARDIO EXERCISE	TIME	CALORIES BURNED

STRETCHING YES ☐ NO ☐

NUTRITION FAT BUDGET _____ FIBER GOAL _____

	FAT GRAMS	FIBER GRAMS
Breakfast:		
Snack:		
Lunch:		
Snack:		
Dinner:		
Notes: **Totals:**		

FOOD GROUP SERVINGS

Fruits ○ ○ ○ ○ ○
Vegetables ○ ○ ○ ○
Calcium-Rich ○ ○ ○
Protein-Rich ○ ○ ○ ○
Breads/Grains ○ ○ ○ ○ ○ ○ ○ ○
Water ○ ○ ○ ○ ○ ○ ○ ○

𝕵ood 𝕵act

Americans spend more than $800 million a year on laxatives to treat constipation when a few tablespoons a day of raw wheat bran might do the trick.

Week 7 TUESDAY DATE

CARDIO EXERCISE | TIME | CALORIES BURNED

STRETCHING YES ☐ NO ☐

NUTRITION FAT BUDGET _____ FIBER GOAL _____

	FAT GRAMS	FIBER GRAMS
Breakfast:		
Snack:		
Lunch:		
Snack:		
Dinner:		
Notes: **Totals:**		

FOOD GROUP SERVINGS

Fruits ○ ○ ○ ○ ○
Vegetables ○ ○ ○ ○
Calcium-Rich ○ ○ ○
Protein-Rich ○ ○ ○ ○
Breads/Grains ○ ○ ○ ○ ○ ○ ○ ○ ○
Water ○ ○ ○ ○ ○ ○ ○ ○

Food Fact

Aim to overshoot your Fiber Goal because the amount of dietary fiber listed on food labels tends to be overestimated. No one's trying to cheat you; it's just that fiber content is difficult to measure in a lab.

Week 7 WEDNESDAY DATE _____

CARDIO EXERCISE | TIME | CALORIES BURNED

_____ | _____ | _____

STRETCHING YES ___ NO ___

NUTRITION FAT BUDGET _____ FIBER GOAL _____

	FAT GRAMS	FIBER GRAMS
Breakfast:		
Snack:		
Lunch:		
Snack:		
Dinner:		
Notes: **Totals:**		

FOOD GROUP SERVINGS

Fruits ○ ○ ○ ○ ○
Vegetables ○ ○ ○ ○
Calcium-Rich ○ ○ ○
Protein-Rich ○ ○ ○ ○
Breads/Grains ○ ○ ○ ○ ○ ○ ○ ○ ○
Water ○ ○ ○ ○ ○ ○ ○

Fitness Tip

If you have time at the end of your workout, use your stretching routine as a time to relax and unwind. If you've just done a tough toning session or step aerobics video, stretching can be a great transition back into your day.

Week 7 THURSDAY   DATE [ ]

CARDIO EXERCISE   TIME   CALORIES BURNED
[ ]   [ ]   [ ]

STRETCHING   YES [ ]   NO [ ]

NUTRITION   FAT BUDGET _____   FIBER GOAL _____

	FAT GRAMS	FIBER GRAMS
Breakfast:		
Snack:		
Lunch:		
Snack:		
Dinner:		
Notes: **Totals:**		

FOOD GROUP SERVINGS

Fruits   ○ ○ ○ ○ ○
Vegetables   ○ ○ ○ ○
Calcium-Rich   ○ ○ ○
Protein-Rich   ○ ○ ○ ○
Breads/Grains   ○ ○ ○ ○ ○ ○ ○ ○ ○
Water   ○ ○ ○ ○ ○ ○ ○ ○

Food Fact
If a food label mentions that high-fiber foods may reduce cancer risk, the product is a good choice. The government will allow a company to make health claims only if the product is also low in fat.

Week 7 FRIDAY

DATE

CARDIO EXERCISE

TIME

CALORIES BURNED

STRETCHING YES NO

NUTRITION FAT BUDGET _____ FIBER GOAL _____

	FAT GRAMS	FIBER GRAMS
Breakfast:		
Snack:		
Lunch:		
Snack:		
Dinner:		
Notes: **Totals:**		

FOOD GROUP SERVINGS

Fruits   ○ ○ ○ ○ ○
Vegetables   ○ ○ ○ ○
Calcium-Rich   ○ ○ ○
Protein-Rich   ○ ○ ○ ○
Breads/Grains   ○ ○ ○ ○ ○ ○ ○ ○ ○
Water   ○ ○ ○ ○ ○ ○ ○ ○

Fitness Tip

Remember that walking, cycling, and weight lifting aren't the only types of activities that will help you lose fat. You can burn extra calories just by being more active during the day—raking leaves, vacuuming the living room, mowing the lawn.

Week 7 SATURDAY   DATE

CARDIO EXERCISE   TIME   CALORIES BURNED

STRETCHING   YES   NO

NUTRITION   FAT BUDGET _____   FIBER GOAL _____

	FAT GRAMS	FIBER GRAMS
Breakfast:		
Snack:		
Lunch:		
Snack:		
Dinner:		
Notes: **Totals:**		

FOOD GROUP SERVINGS

Fruits   ○ ○ ○ ○ ○
Vegetables   ○ ○ ○ ○
Calcium-Rich   ○ ○ ○
Protein-Rich   ○ ○ ○ ○
Breads/Grains   ○ ○ ○ ○ ○ ○ ○ ○ ○
Water   ○ ○ ○ ○ ○ ○ ○ ○

Food Fact

It's not a problem for most of us, but you *can* get too much fiber. Eating more than 50 grams of fiber per day is associated with diarrhea and bloating and possibly a reduced absorption of minerals such as zinc and iron.

Week 7 SUNDAY

DATE

CARDIO EXERCISE

TIME

CALORIES BURNED

STRETCHING YES ☐ NO ☐

NUTRITION FAT BUDGET _____ FIBER GOAL _____

	FAT GRAMS	FIBER GRAMS
Breakfast:		
Snack:		
Lunch:		
Snack:		
Dinner:		
Notes: **Totals:**		

FOOD GROUP SERVINGS

Fruits	○ ○ ○ ○ ○
Vegetables	○ ○ ○ ○
Calcium-Rich	○ ○ ○
Protein-Rich	○ ○ ○ ○
Breads/Grains	○ ○ ○ ○ ○ ○ ○ ○ ○
Water	○ ○ ○ ○ ○ ○ ○ ○ ○

Food Fact

If a package says "good source of fiber," the food must have at least 2.5 grams of fiber per serving. "High-fiber" foods need 5 grams or more. Fi-Bar fat-free granola bars can't make either claim; each bar has only 2 grams of fiber.

WEEK IN REVIEW

TONING

DAYS [ ]   DID YOU MEET THE GOAL? _____

NOTES _____

_____

CARDIO EXERCISE

DAYS [ ]   CALORIES [ ]   DID YOU MEET THE GOALS? _____

NOTES _____

_____

WEIGHT [ ]

NUTRITION

DAYS UNDER FAT BUDGET [ ]   FOOD FOCUS RATING, 1–5 [ ]

Take a few moments to reflect on all the progress you've made since Week 1. What's been your greatest success? Where do you need to improve? Make the most of your final three weeks.
— Kathy

WATER
AND TRICEPS

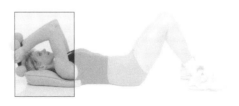

Water

Whenever I step onto an airplane—well, you should just *feel* how heavy my carry-on bag is. It's not that I've overpacked; it's my water bottles! I never travel without at least two of them. Drinking lots of water saves me from getting dehydrated on the plane and feeling jet-lagged when I get off.

There's absolutely no substance on earth more important than water. You could skimp on protein or fiber if you had to, but you just can't survive without water. It's even more vital when you exercise. Your muscle tissue is about 75 percent water, and even a tiny deficit can profoundly affect how your body performs. Your blood is about 90 percent water. When you don't drink enough, your body becomes less efficient at transporting nutrients to your muscles and carrying away waste products. Your body also uses water to digest your food, lubricate your joints, and create a protective cushion around your organs and tissues.

This week your goal is to drink 8 glasses of water on days that you don't exercise, and at least 9 glasses on your workout days. You've probably heard these numbers before, but did you ever wonder where they came from? Here's a rundown: The average person loses 10 cups of water per day—2 cups to sweating and evaporation, 2 cups to breathing, and 6 cups to waste removal. You can replace up to 2 cups through the water in the foods you eat, but you have to make up the remaining 8 cups by drinking fluids, water being the best choice. But on the days you work out, you need much *more* water—anywhere from 9 to 13 cups a day, depending on how active you are. For every half hour you exercise, add at least an extra cup of water.

Throughout the day, don't rely on thirst to tell you when to drink. By the time your brain says, "Hey, water—*now!*" you probably are already dehydrated. You can prevent this situation by drinking all day long. The best strategy is to keep a water bottle within reach during the day, whether it's sitting on your desk at work or on a table at home. You'll drink without even noticing, and before you know it, your bottle will be empty. It's a lot easier and more efficient than constantly heading to the drinking fountain or the kitchen.

Be extra sure to keep a water bottle handy during your workouts. There are some terrific fanny packs that hold water bottles—they're great for walking or hiking. Another option is the CamelBak, a pouch of water that you wear on your back like a backpack; you suck the water through a tube that hangs down from your shoulder. It's great for cycling or walking. If you have a treadmill, stairclimber, or stationary bike at home, you can buy a plastic water bottle holder that fits right on the console.

What if you don't like the taste of water? That's easily rectified. Your fluids don't have to come entirely from plain water itself. Juice counts, milk counts—just about any decaffeinated or nonalcoholic beverage counts. But water is the best choice because it's calorie-free. Orange juice is 90 percent water, but if you drank 8 glasses a day, that would be 720 calories! One of my favorite tricks is to mix water with a tablespoon or two of cranberry or apple juice. That way it's more palatable and you save calories.

Triceps

What can you do about flabby arms? Plenty! Often the "flab" at the back of the arm is really just untrained muscle. Most of us *do* store some fat in that area, but you can make a tremendous difference just by training your triceps, your rear upper arm muscle.

Most of us have relatively weak triceps because this muscle doesn't get much action on a day-to-day basis. You use your triceps every time you push—whether you're pushing away from a table or pushing a box up onto a high shelf. But think about it: How much time do you spend pushing something heavy enough to give you muscle tone?

Triceps exercises will give your arms that sculpted shape without making them look bulky. Meanwhile, you'll be doing your elbow joints a favor. With most of us, the triceps are overpowered by the biceps, the muscle at the *front* of the upper arm. This combination of weak triceps and strong biceps can leave you more prone to elbow injuries. The exercises in my program will get your triceps up to par and give you firm, toned arms you'll be proud of.

Muscle Basics

Your *triceps brachii,* as it's formally called, is a three-headed muscle that covers the rear of your upper arm. All three heads—the lateral (outer), medial (inner), and long—work together to straighten your arm.

Week 8: The Plan

Workouts This Week: 2–3

Sets per Exercise: 2–3

Reps per Set: 12–15

Reps per Abdominal Set: 15–20

Toning Focus: Triceps

TONING EXERCISE	PAGE
1. French Press	248
2. Triceps Kickback	250
3. Seated Biceps Curl	252
4. Push-up	238
5. One-Arm Row	234
6. Reverse Curl	212
7. Cross Crunch	214
8. Backward Lunge	222
9. Hamstring Curl	232
10. Standing Side Lift	228
11. Inner Thigh Pull	230
12. Toe Raise	258

Cardio Exercise

Calories to Burn: 700+

Total Days: 3–4+

Food Focus: Water

Goal: At least 8 glasses of water per day

TONING DAY 1

DATE _____

FOCUS: **Triceps**

	SETS	REPS	WEIGHT
1. French Press			
2. Triceps Kickback			
3. Seated Biceps Curl			
4. Push-up			
5. One-Arm Row			
6. Reverse Curl			
7. Cross Crunch			
8. Backward Lunge			
9. Hamstring Curl			
10. Standing Side Lift			
11. Inner Thigh Pull			
12. Toe Raise			

TONING DAY 2

DATE _____

FOCUS: **Triceps**

	SETS	REPS	WEIGHT
1. French Press			
2. Triceps Kickback			
3. Seated Biceps Curl			
4. Push-up			
5. One-Arm Row			
6. Reverse Curl			
7. Cross Crunch			
8. Backward Lunge			
9. Hamstring Curl			
10. Standing Side Lift			
11. Inner Thigh Pull			
12. Toe Raise			

TONING DAY 3

DATE _____

FOCUS: **Triceps**

	SETS	REPS	WEIGHT
1. French Press			
2. Triceps Kickback			
3. Seated Biceps Curl			
4. Push-up			
5. One-Arm Row			
6. Reverse Curl			
7. Cross Crunch			
8. Backward Lunge			
9. Hamstring Curl			
10. Standing Side Lift			
11. Inner Thigh Pull			
12. Toe Raise			

Week 8 MONDAY DATE

CARDIO EXERCISE | TIME | CALORIES BURNED

STRETCHING YES [ ] NO [ ]

NUTRITION FAT BUDGET _____ WATER GOAL _____

	FAT GRAMS	CUPS OF WATER
Breakfast:		
Snack:		
Lunch:		
Snack:		
Dinner:		
Notes: **Totals:**		

FOOD GROUP SERVINGS

Fruits ○ ○ ○ ○ ○
Vegetables ○ ○ ○ ○
Calcium-Rich ○ ○ ○
Protein-Rich ○ ○ ○ ○
Breads/Grains ○ ○ ○ ○ ○ ○ ○ ○ ○
Water ○ ○ ○ ○ ○ ○ ○ ○

Food Fact

Some people are afraid to drink water during a workout or a 10k run because they think it will give them cramps. But just the opposite is true. *Dehydration* is what causes cramps. Don't skimp on the water!

Week 8 TUESDAY

DATE

CARDIO EXERCISE

TIME

CALORIES BURNED

STRETCHING YES ☐ NO ☐

NUTRITION FAT BUDGET _____ WATER GOAL _____

	FAT GRAMS	CUPS OF WATER
Breakfast:		
Snack:		
Lunch:		
Snack:		
Dinner:		
Notes: **Totals:**		

FOOD GROUP SERVINGS

Fruits ○ ○ ○ ○ ○
Vegetables ○ ○ ○ ○
Calcium-Rich ○ ○ ○
Protein-Rich ○ ○ ○ ○
Breads/Grains ○ ○ ○ ○ ○ ○ ○ ○ ○
Water ○ ○ ○ ○ ○ ○ ○ ○ ○

Food Fact

Dehydration isn't something that just happens over the course of a day. You can create a water deficit in your body over a period of days or even several weeks. You can also become dehydrated during a single workout.

Week 8 WEDNESDAY DATE

CARDIO EXERCISE   TIME   CALORIES BURNED

STRETCHING   YES   NO

NUTRITION   FAT BUDGET _____   WATER GOAL _____

		FAT GRAMS	CUPS OF WATER
Breakfast:			
Snack:			
Lunch:			
Snack:			
Dinner:			
Notes:	**Totals:**		

FOOD GROUP SERVINGS

Fruits ○ ○ ○ ○ ○
Vegetables ○ ○ ○ ○
Calcium-Rich ○ ○ ○
Protein-Rich ○ ○ ○ ○
Breads/Grains ○ ○ ○ ○ ○ ○ ○ ○ ○
Water ○ ○ ○ ○ ○ ○ ○ ○ ○

Fitness Tip

Strength training just might help you lose weight and keep it off. If you add enough muscle to your body, it's possible that you'll rev up your metabolism, although research has yet to prove this definitively.

Week 8 THURSDAY   DATE [ ]

CARDIO EXERCISE   TIME   CALORIES BURNED
[ ]   [ ]   [ ]

STRETCHING   YES [ ]   NO [ ]

NUTRITION   FAT BUDGET _____   WATER GOAL _____

	FAT GRAMS	CUPS OF WATER
Breakfast:		
Snack:		
Lunch:		
Snack:		
Dinner:		
Notes: **Totals:**		

FOOD GROUP SERVINGS

Fruits ○ ○ ○ ○ ○
Vegetables ○ ○ ○ ○
Calcium-Rich ○ ○ ○
Protein-Rich ○ ○ ○ ○
Breads/Grains ○ ○ ○ ○ ○ ○ ○ ○ ○
Water ○ ○ ○ ○ ○ ○ ○ ○ ○

Food Fact

Sports drinks aren't just a bunch of hype. The carbohydrates in them will help you ward off fatigue during a workout, especially if you're exercising for more than an hour. Plus, if you like the taste, you might drink more fluid than if you were drinking plain water.

Week 8 FRIDAY DATE [ ]

CARDIO EXERCISE TIME CALORIES BURNED
[ ] [ ] [ ]

STRETCHING YES [ ] NO [ ]

NUTRITION FAT BUDGET _____ WATER GOAL _____

	FAT GRAMS	CUPS OF WATER
Breakfast:		
Snack:		
Lunch:		
Snack:		
Dinner:		
Notes: Totals:		

FOOD GROUP SERVINGS

Fruits   ○ ○ ○ ○ ○
Vegetables   ○ ○ ○ ○
Calcium-Rich   ○ ○ ○
Protein-Rich   ○ ○ ○ ○
Breads/Grains   ○ ○ ○ ○ ○ ○ ○ ○ ○
Water   ○ ○ ○ ○ ○ ○ ○ ○

Fitness Tip

During your toning workouts, remember to breathe. I'm serious! Breathing sounds like second nature, but it's something people tend to forget about when lifting weights. Holding your breath can increase your blood pressure and zap your energy.

Week 8 SATURDAY   DATE ____

CARDIO EXERCISE | TIME | CALORIES BURNED

| | | |

STRETCHING YES ☐   NO ☐

NUTRITION Fat Budget ____ Water Goal ____

	FAT GRAMS	CUPS OF WATER
Breakfast:		
Snack:		
Lunch:		
Snack:		
Dinner:		
Notes: **Totals:**		

FOOD GROUP SERVINGS

Fruits ○○○○○
Vegetables ○○○○
Calcium-Rich ○○○
Protein-Rich ○○○○
Breads/Grains ○○○○○○○○○
Water ○○○○○○○○○

Food Fact

The simplest way to tell if you're drinking enough is to check the color and quantity of your urine. If it's clear and plentiful, you're doing fine. If it's dark and scanty, you need to drink more. If you're taking vitamin supplements, your urine may be dark, so in that case, volume is a better indicator than color.

Week 8 SUNDAY

DATE

CARDIO EXERCISE

TIME

CALORIES BURNED

STRETCHING YES NO

NUTRITION FAT BUDGET _____ WATER GOAL _____

	FAT GRAMS	CUPS OF WATER
Breakfast:		
Snack:		
Lunch:		
Snack:		
Dinner:		
Notes: **Totals:**		

FOOD GROUP SERVINGS

Fruits ○ ○ ○ ○ ○
Vegetables ○ ○ ○ ○
Calcium-Rich ○ ○ ○
Protein-Rich ○ ○ ○ ○
Breads/Grains ○ ○ ○ ○ ○ ○ ○ ○ ○
Water ○ ○ ○ ○ ○ ○ ○ ○

Food Fact

By the time your brain signals thirst, you may have lost 1 percent of your body weight. If you're working out, a 2 percent loss can slow you down by 10 percent to 15 percent. It's not uncommon to lose a few pounds during a tough workout. To rehydrate, consume 16 ounces of fluid for every pound lost during exercise.

WEEK IN REVIEW

TONING

DAYS [   ]   DID YOU MEET THE GOAL? _____

NOTES _____

_____

CARDIO EXERCISE

DAYS [   ]   CALORIES [   ]   DID YOU MEET THE GOALS? _____

NOTES _____

_____

WEIGHT [   ]

NUTRITION

DAYS UNDER FAT BUDGET [   ]   FOOD FOCUS RATING, 1–5 [   ]

Whenever you feel yourself becoming a little tense or anxious, try my favorite strategy: Jake a five minute break. Just five minutes spent sitting quietly can help you put perspective on the events of the day.

Kathy

VITAMINS AND MINERALS AND BICEPS

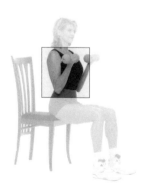

Vitamins and Minerals

NUTRITION GOAL RECAP

This week, maximize the vitamins and minerals you get from your diet by eating plenty of fruits, vegetables, and whole grains. For insurance, take a multivitamin/mineral supplement every day.

Back in the early 1980s, when high-impact, high-intensity aerobics was the big craze, I'd come home from teaching a bunch of classes and just collapse on the couch from exhaustion. Turns out, it wasn't the workouts that were killing me; it was my diet. "I don't even know how you're *moving*," my doctor told me. "You're extremely anemic." A few years earlier I'd stopped eating meat, and I wasn't doing anything to compensate for the lost iron.

The experience was a real lesson to me. You can't just yank a food group from your diet and expect your body to resume business as usual. Eventually, you'll end up with a vitamin or mineral shortage that could compromise your health. Even though we use tiny amounts of these nutrients—a day's worth of vitamins wouldn't fill one-fourth of a teaspoon—vitamins and minerals are utterly precious. They're involved in every one of your body's functions; they help build, maintain, and repair your body's tissues, and they aid in the crucial process of converting foods into energy. Vegetarian diets can be perfectly healthy, but only if you take special care to make up for the lost nutrients. The same goes for low-fat, low-calorie diets. When you're trying to lose weight, you tend to focus on the *benefits* of cutting out certain foods; but you also need to take a look at what might be missing.

The typical American diet is missing a lot. This is partly due to dieting, but it's also due to our affinity for processed foods. We've substituted them for whole grains, fresh fruits, and vegetables, and as a result, saddled ourselves with nutrient deficiencies. Surveys show that 90 percent of Americans get half or less of the recommended amount of chromium, a mineral that's important for regulating blood sugar levels. We also tend to be low in magnesium, which helps metabolize energy, develop muscle, and maintain healthy bones. When it comes to iron, up to 80 percent of exercising women—and 20 percent of women in general—may fall short. As I learned, the consequences of iron deficiency can be significant: Your tissues become starved for oxygen, you tire easily, and you tend to lose concentration. (I've gone back to eating meat and poultry, but I stick to extra-lean cuts.)

The list goes on and on. What's the solution? As I've mentioned throughout the book, we all need to cut back on processed foods and eat more fruits, vegetables, whole grains, and low-fat dairy products. Of course, most of us lead fast-paced lives that don't always allow for the perfect balanced diet, despite our best intentions. That's why I take a multivitamin/mineral supplement every day. I consider it a form of health insurance. Evidence is piling up that certain vitamins and minerals can bolster your immune system and help prevent cancer, heart disease, and premature aging. I don't want to risk missing out on these potential benefits.

Your goal this week is to maximize the vitamins and minerals you get from your diet by eating plenty of fruits, vegetables, and whole grains. I also recommend taking a multivitamin/mineral supplement every day. It's one of the easiest healthy habits to adopt! You don't need to buy a bottle of those high-priced megavitamins; your body can use only so much of each nutrient, anyway. In general, 100 percent of the daily value for each nutrient is sufficient—after all, this is just to *supplement* what comes naturally from food. Exceptions to this rule are the antioxidant nutrients—vitamin C, vitamin E, and beta-carotene—which might be beneficial in doses several times larger than the current U.S. RDA levels. As I mentioned in Week 6, you might also consider a separate calcium supplement. (Many regular multivitamin/mineral supplements don't contain much calcium.)

Supplements can give you a sense of security about your health, but don't use them to compensate for poor eating habits. Most nutrient experts agree that food is still the best source of vitamins and minerals.

Biceps

Even though I've been weight training for twenty-five years, it wasn't until six months ago that I started to pay special attention to my biceps. One day I looked in the mirror and realized: My arms are skinny! People these days are so concerned with being thin, thin, thin. But the truth is, ultra-thin arms will only make you look frail. By focusing on your biceps, you can project a much more vigorous, youthful image.

But you won't just notice the changes in the mirror. You'll see the results of your biceps training every time you lift your kids or carry a heavy grocery bag in your arms. Now that I've been focusing on my biceps, I can lift things that were too heavy for me ten years ago! I've even gained enough arm strength to do two full chin-ups. My goal is to do six. I'm sure I'll get there one of these days.

One last word on biceps: Some women are afraid to train these muscles for fear they'll develop bulky arms. Believe me, it won't happen. Building huge muscles requires plenty of testosterone (the hormone men have a lot of) and a workout routine with extremely heavy weights. You don't have to worry about either one.

Muscle Basics

Your biceps are really two muscles: your *biceps brachii* and your *brachialis*. The brachialis is the larger and deeper of the two; the biceps brachii sits on top and gives the front of your upper arm much of its shape. You use these muscles anytime you pick up an object or pull something toward you.

Week 9: The Plan

Workouts This Week: 2–3

Sets per Exercise: 2–3

Reps per Set: 12–15

Reps per Abdominal Set: 15–20

Toning Focus: Biceps

TONING EXERCISE	PAGE
1. Seated Biceps Curl	252
2. Concentration Curl	254
3. French Press	248
4. Chest Flye	240
5. Rear Raise	246
6. Front Raise	244
7. Squat	226
8. Hip Lift	220
9. Inner Thigh Pull	230
10. Standing Side Lift	228
11. Crunch	210
12. Back Extension	216

Cardio Exercise
Calories to Burn: 750+
Total Days: 3–5+

Food Focus: Vitamins and Minerals
Goal: Take a supplement every day

TONING DAY 1

DATE _____

FOCUS: **Biceps**

	SETS	REPS	WEIGHT
1. Seated Biceps Curl			
2. Concentration Curl			
3. French Press			
4. Chest Flye			
5. Rear Raise			
6. Front Raise			
7. Squat			
8. Hip Lift			
9. Inner Thigh Pull			
10. Standing Side Lift			
11. Crunch			
12. Back Extension			

TONING DAY 2

DATE _____

FOCUS: **Biceps**

	SETS	REPS	WEIGHT
1. Seated Biceps Curl			
2. Concentration Curl			
3. French Press			
4. Chest Flye			
5. Rear Raise			
6. Front Raise			
7. Squat			
8. Hip Lift			
9. Inner Thigh Pull			
10. Standing Side Lift			
11. Crunch			
12. Back Extension			

TONING DAY 3

DATE _____

FOCUS: **Biceps**

	SETS	REPS	WEIGHT
1. Seated Biceps Curl			
2. Concentration Curl			
3. French Press			
4. Chest Flye			
5. Rear Raise			
6. Front Raise			
7. Squat			
8. Hip Lift			
9. Inner Thigh Pull			
10. Standing Side Lift			
11. Crunch			
12. Back Extension			

Week 9 MONDAY

DATE [ ]

CARDIO EXERCISE | TIME | CALORIES BURNED

[ ] | [ ] | [ ]

STRETCHING YES [ ] NO [ ]

NUTRITION FAT BUDGET _____ TOOK SUPPLEMENT _____

FAT GRAMS

	FAT GRAMS
Breakfast:	
Snack:	
Lunch:	
Snack:	
Dinner:	
Notes: **Totals:**	

FOOD GROUP SERVINGS

Fruits ○ ○ ○ ○ ○
Vegetables ○ ○ ○ ○
Calcium-Rich ○ ○ ○
Protein-Rich ○ ○ ○ ○
Breads/Grains ○ ○ ○ ○ ○ ○ ○ ○ ○
Water ○ ○ ○ ○ ○ ○ ○ ○

Food Fact

It's tough to meet all your nutritional needs without at least one serving of dark green leafy vegetables every day. They provide folic acid, vitamin A, calcium, iron, magnesium, and potassium. Still, 80 percent of women often go four whole days without a single serving.

Week 9 TUESDAY

DATE [ ]

CARDIO EXERCISE

TIME

CALORIES BURNED

[ ] [ ] [ ]

STRETCHING YES [ ] NO [ ]

NUTRITION FAT BUDGET _____ TOOK SUPPLEMENT _____

FAT GRAMS

	FAT GRAMS
Breakfast:	
Snack:	
Lunch:	
Snack:	
Dinner:	
Notes: **Totals:**	

FOOD GROUP SERVINGS

Fruits ○ ○ ○ ○ ○
Vegetables ○ ○ ○ ○
Calcium-Rich ○ ○ ○
Protein-Rich ○ ○ ○ ○
Breads/Grains ○ ○ ○ ○ ○ ○ ○ ○ ○
Water ○ ○ ○ ○ ○ ○ ○ ○

Food Fact

Avocados are 88 percent fat, but don't be scared off by them entirely! A single avocado supplies one-fourth your daily need for magnesium, one-half the folic acid, and one-fourth the vitamin A, plus lots of B vitamins, iron, and trace minerals.

Week 9   WEDNESDAY DATE

CARDIO EXERCISE   TIME   CALORIES BURNED

STRETCHING YES [ ]   NO [ ]

NUTRITION FAT BUDGET _____ TOOK SUPPLEMENT _____

FAT GRAMS

	FAT GRAMS
Breakfast:	
Snack:	
Lunch:	
Snack:	
Dinner:	
Notes:	**Totals:**

FOOD GROUP SERVINGS

Fruits   ○ ○ ○ ○ ○
Vegetables   ○ ○ ○ ○
Calcium-Rich   ○ ○ ○
Protein-Rich   ○ ○ ○ ○
Breads/Grains   ○ ○ ○ ○ ○ ○ ○ ○ ○
Water   ○ ○ ○ ○ ○ ○ ○ ○

Fitness Tip

"Maintain Your Bone Mass"—that's not a headline you're likely to see on a magazine cover. After all, bone health isn't the sexiest topic around. Nevertheless, if you don't overload your bones by lifting weight, they have no incentive to stay strong.

Week 9 THURSDAY   DATE

CARDIO EXERCISE   TIME   CALORIES BURNED

STRETCHING   YES   NO

NUTRITION   FAT BUDGET _____   TOOK SUPPLEMENT _____

FAT GRAMS

	FAT GRAMS
Breakfast:	
Snack:	
Lunch:	
Snack:	
Dinner:	
Notes: **Totals:**	

FOOD GROUP SERVINGS

Fruits   ○ ○ ○ ○ ○
Vegetables   ○ ○ ○ ○
Calcium-Rich ○ ○ ○
Protein-Rich ○ ○ ○ ○
Breads/Grains ○ ○ ○ ○ ○ ○ ○ ○ ○
Water   ○ ○ ○ ○ ○ ○ ○ ○

Food Fact

Buy fruits and vegetables that are fresh or frozen and, as a last resort, canned. The high temperatures involved in canning can destroy some vitamins. Also, you can maximize your vitamin intake by cooking or steaming your vegetables until just tender in the least amount of water possible.

Week 9 FRIDAY

DATE [ ]

CARDIO EXERCISE

TIME | CALORIES BURNED

STRETCHING YES [ ]   NO [ ]

NUTRITION FAT BUDGET _____ TOOK SUPPLEMENT _____

FAT GRAMS

	FAT GRAMS
Breakfast:	
Snack:	
Lunch:	
Snack:	
Dinner:	
Notes:	**Totals:**

FOOD GROUP SERVINGS

Fruits   ○ ○ ○ ○ ○
Vegetables   ○ ○ ○ ○
Calcium-Rich   ○ ○ ○
Protein-Rich   ○ ○ ○ ○
Breads/Grains   ○ ○ ○ ○ ○ ○ ○ ○ ○
Water   ○ ○ ○ ○ ○ ○ ○ ○

Fitness Tip

You probably know that cardiovascular exercise can lower your blood pressure, cholesterol level, and risk for heart disease and diabetes. But did you know that moderate cardio exercise can also reduce stress and leave you less susceptible to colds and the flu?

Week 9 SATURDAY DATE

CARDIO EXERCISE TIME CALORIES BURNED

STRETCHING YES NO

NUTRITION FAT BUDGET _____ TOOK SUPPLEMENT _____

FAT GRAMS

Breakfast:	
Snack:	
Lunch:	
Snack:	
Dinner:	
Notes:	**Totals:**

FOOD GROUP SERVINGS

Fruits ○ ○ ○ ○ ○
Vegetables ○ ○ ○ ○
Calcium-Rich ○ ○ ○
Protein-Rich ○ ○ ○ ○
Breads/Grains ○ ○ ○ ○ ○ ○ ○ ○ ○
Water ○ ○ ○ ○ ○ ○ ○ ○

Food Fact

Vitamins don't directly give you energy—they don't have any calories. However, vitamin deficiencies can make you feel lethargic. So, if you're short on some vitamins, increasing your intake may help you metabolize energy more efficiently.

Week 9 SUNDAY

DATE

CARDIO EXERCISE

TIME

CALORIES BURNED

STRETCHING YES ☐ NO ☐

NUTRITION FAT BUDGET _____ TOOK SUPPLEMENT _____

FAT GRAMS

	FAT GRAMS
Breakfast:	
Snack:	
Lunch:	
Snack:	
Dinner:	
Notes: **Totals:**	

FOOD GROUP SERVINGS

Fruits ○ ○ ○ ○ ○
Vegetables ○ ○ ○ ○
Calcium-Rich ○ ○ ○
Protein-Rich ○ ○ ○ ○
Breads/Grains ○ ○ ○ ○ ○ ○ ○ ○ ○
Water ○ ○ ○ ○ ○ ○ ○ ○ ○

Food Fact

Surveys show that women are low in iron and zinc. Fish and poultry products provide adequate protein, but they provide only about half as much zinc and iron as lean red meats. Great sources of these minerals include lean sirloin cuts such as tenderloin, top sirloin, round steak, and lean roast beef.

WEEK IN REVIEW

TONING

DAYS [ ]   DID YOU MEET THE GOAL? _____

NOTES _____

_____

CARDIO EXERCISE

DAYS [ ]   CALORIES [ ]   DID YOU MEET THE GOALS? _____

NOTES _____

_____

WEIGHT [ ]

NUTRITION

DAYS UNDER FAT BUDGET [ ]   FOOD FOCUS RATING, 1–5 [ ]

In some ways, this book is like a video: you can refer to it over and over.
There's no limit to how much you can learn about your body!
Kathy.

SUGAR AND
CALVES AND SHINS

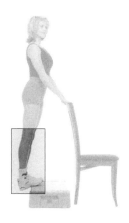

Sugar

NUTRITION GOAL RECAP

This week, watch your sugar intake and give yourself a point in the Low-Sugar Carb column each time you choose a low-sugar food instead of a high-sugar item. As in Week 4 (Quality Starches), I'm not giving you a numerical goal.

Back in Week 4, you focused on eating more complex carbohydrates such as whole wheat bread, brown rice, fruits, and vegetables. Well, this week we're going to focus on the flip side of the carbohydrate discussion: cutting back on added sugar. In other words, rather than concentrate on eating more whole grains, you'll focus on eating fewer sweets. It's just a different approach to the same ultimate goal.

Since many food labels don't list the number of carbohydrate grams that come from added sugar (it's not a government requirement), it can be tough to accurately estimate how much sugar you're eating. Still, the list of ingredients offers clues about how much sugar is in a product. The higher "sugar" is listed, the more sugar the product contains. If sugar is listed in the top three ingredients of a product, you're better off with an alternative brand.

This week, pay attention to labels, and give yourself a point in the Low-Sugar Carb column every time you consciously replace your usual high-sugar food with a low-sugar substitute. For instance, if you normally eat Kellogg's Apple Jacks (51 percent sugar!), give yourself a point for eating Kellogg's Rice Krispies (8 percent sugar). Pay special attention to snacks, which tend to be high in sugar.

Beware of hidden sugars! We all know that cookies, cakes, candy, and ice cream are loaded with sugar. But there's often plenty of sugar in foods like ketchup, salad dressing, peanut butter, and canned soups. Dannon vanilla yogurt has more added sugar than a Mr. Goodbar! It's no big deal if you're eating foods like these in small amounts, but if you eat yogurt every day for breakfast or use salad dressing every day at lunch, make sure your choices are low in sugar.

You might be wondering: Is sugar really so bad for you? Unlike fat, sugar has not been directly implicated in any disease other than tooth decay. However, sugar—in the massive quantities that Americans consume it—can contribute to obesity, which in turn can lead to heart disease and cancer. Human beings have always loved sweets. In fact, studies show we're *born* with a sweet tooth—the sweeter a liquid, the more babies want to drink it. However, only in recent decades have we gone sugar crazy. In 1840, the typical American consumed 4 teaspoons of sugar a day, mostly in homemade jams and desserts. Today, we've shot up to 43 teaspoons a day! Added sugars now make up nearly 20 percent of our total calories, up from 11 percent early in the century.

The sugar itself is less harmful than the absence of healthier foods. We've replaced wholesome, complex carbs with nutritionally worthless ones. As a result of eating more sugar, we're getting less fiber and fewer vitamins and minerals. We're also setting ourselves up to gain weight. All carbs have 4 calories per gram, but as I mentioned in Week 4, sugar doesn't make you feel nearly as full as, say, pasta or bread. You can easily spend your whole day's calorie budget on one candy bar, a handful of chocolate chip cookies, and hot fudge sundae—hardly a satisfying quantity of food. Besides, eating sugar will only lead you to crave more sugar.

By the same token, once you start weaning yourself from sugar, you'll find yourself less drawn to it. In fact, high-sugar foods may start to taste too sweet to you. Now that I eat plain, nonfat yogurt topped with raisins, yogurt with lots of sugar tastes awful to me.

You're probably wondering about sugar substitutes like aspartame (NutraSweet). Are they okay to eat? Well, aspartame hasn't been shown to be harmful in moderation, and a diet soda is a better choice than a regular soda because you'll save the calories. But ultimately, diet soda has the same problem as regular soda: There's nothing good in it for you!

SUGAR BY ANY OTHER NAME . . .

When you read labels, look for more than "sugar." The added sugar in foods goes by other aliases, including "corn syrup," "sucrose," and "maltodextrin." Here is the ingredients list for a Fi-Bar fat-free blueberry granola bar. The added sugars are highlighted.

INGREDIENTS: GRANOLA (RICE, TOASTED ROLLED WHEAT, TOASTED ROLLED BARLEY, **HONEY, SUCROSE,** MALT, SALT), **CORN SYRUP,** APPLES, **SUCROSE,** BLUEBERRIES, DATES, ACACIA GUM, MODIFIED OAT FLOUR, FIGS, **HIGH FRUCTOSE CORN SYRUP,** WATER, **HONEY,** NONFAT MILK, GLYCERINE, GELLAN GUM, MODIFIED FOOD STARCH, CARAMEL COLOR, SODIUM CITRATE, NATURAL FLAVOR, SALT, MALIC ACID, TARTARIC ACID.

Calves and Shins

Last—but definitely not least—we come to the lower leg. Over the years I've developed strong calf muscles, first from marathon running and more recently from walking and hiking. Still, I feel it's important to challenge my calves with the kind of overload they just don't get out on the trails. Calf exercises give my legs extra power. They'll do the same for you.

Some people have long, narrow calf muscles, while others have shorter, wider ones. No matter how *your* calf muscles are shaped, the exercises in my program will give your lower legs that distinctive curve and muscular look.

Why bother training your shin muscles? After all, most people don't go around thinking, "If only I had sexy shins . . ." The fact is, you need strong shins for muscular balance. You train the front and back of your arms, the front and back of your torso, and the front and back of your thighs. The same principle applies to your lower legs. By balancing your calf and shin muscles, you'll help keep your ankles healthy and help prevent the shin pain that sometimes comes from running and walking.

Muscle Basics

Your calf consists of two muscles: the *soleus* and the *gastrocnemius*. The soleus is the larger muscle and gives your calf most of its size. The gastrocnemius, which has two heads, sits on top of the soleus and provides that diamond shape. Both muscles work together when you point your foot.

You have four shin muscles: the *anterior tibial, posterior tibial, extensor hallucis longus,* and *extensor digitorum longus*. You use these muscles when you pull your foot toward your shin.

Week 10: The Plan

Workouts This Week: 2–3

Sets per Exercise: 2–3

Reps per Set: 12–15

Reps per Abdominal Set: 15–20

Toning Focus: Calves and shins

TONING EXERCISE	PAGE
1. Standing Calf Raise	256
2. Toe Raise	258
3. Backward Lunge	222
4. Hamstring Curl	232
5. Leg Lift	224
6. Cross Crunch	214
7. Back Extension with a Twist	218
8. Push-up	238
9. Seated Back Flye	236
10. Triceps Kickback	250
11. Concentration Curl	254
12. Lateral Raise	242

Cardio Exercise
Calories to Burn: 800+
Total Days: 3–5+

Food Focus: Sugar
Goal: Replace high-sugar foods with low-sugar foods

TONING DAY 1

DATE _____

FOCUS: **Calves and Shins**

	SETS	REPS	WEIGHT
1. Standing Calf Raise			
2. Toe Raise			
3. Backward Lunge			
4. Hamstring Curl			
5. Leg Lift			
6. Cross Crunch			
7. Back Ext. with Twist			
8. Push-up			
9. Seated Back Flye			
10. Triceps Kickback			
11. Concentration Curl			
12. Lateral Raise			

TONING DAY 2

DATE _____

FOCUS: **Calves and Shins**

	SETS	REPS	WEIGHT
1. Standing Calf Raise			
2. Toe Raise			
3. Backward Lunge			
4. Hamstring Curl			
5. Leg Lift			
6. Cross Crunch			
7. Back Ext. with Twist			
8. Push-up			
9. Seated Back Flye			
10. Triceps Kickback			
11. Concentration Curl			
12. Lateral Raise			

TONING DAY 3

DATE _____

Focus: **Calves and Shins**

	SETS	REPS	WEIGHT
1. Standing Calf Raise			
2. Toe Raise			
3. Backward Lunge			
4. Hamstring Curl			
5. Leg Lift			
6. Cross Crunch			
7. Back Ext. with Twist			
8. Push-up			
9. Seated Back Flye			
10. Triceps Kickback			
11. Concentration Curl			
12. Lateral Raise			

Week 10 MONDAY DATE ☐

CARDIO EXERCISE | TIME | CALORIES BURNED

STRETCHING YES ☐ NO ☐

NUTRITION FAT BUDGET _____

	FAT GRAMS	LOW-SUGAR CARB
Breakfast:		
Snack:		
Lunch:		
Snack:		
Dinner:		
Notes: **Totals:**		

FOOD GROUP SERVINGS

Fruits ○ ○ ○ ○ ○
Vegetables ○ ○ ○ ○
Calcium-Rich ○ ○ ○
Protein-Rich ○ ○ ○ ○
Breads/Grains ○ ○ ○ ○ ○ ○ ○ ○ ○
Water ○ ○ ○ ○ ○ ○ ○ ○ ○

Food Fact

Americans average more than 450 cans of regular soda per year. At 5 to 9 teaspoons of sugar per can, that's 2,250 to 4,050 teaspoons of sugar a year from soft drinks alone!

Week 10 TUESDAY   DATE

CARDIO EXERCISE   TIME   CALORIES BURNED

STRETCHING YES ☐   NO ☐

NUTRITION FAT BUDGET _____

	FAT GRAMS	LOW-SUGAR CARB
Breakfast:		
Snack:		
Lunch:		
Snack:		
Dinner:		
Notes: **Totals:**		

FOOD GROUP SERVINGS

Fruits ○ ○ ○ ○ ○
Vegetables ○ ○ ○ ○
Calcium-Rich ○ ○ ○
Protein-Rich ○ ○ ○ ○
Breads/Grains ○ ○ ○ ○ ○ ○ ○ ○ ○
Water ○ ○ ○ ○ ○ ○ ○ ○ ○

Food Fact

Some people are so sensitive to sugar that even one glazed donut can send them on a mood-swing roller coaster. For some people, clinical depression literally vanishes—within a week—when they eliminate sugar.

Week 10 WEDNESDAY DATE _____

CARDIO EXERCISE   TIME   CALORIES BURNED

STRETCHING   YES ____   NO ____

NUTRITION   FAT BUDGET _____

	FAT GRAMS	LOW-SUGAR CARB
Breakfast:		
Snack:		
Lunch:		
Snack:		
Dinner:		
Notes: **Totals:**		

FOOD GROUP SERVINGS

Fruits   ○ ○ ○ ○ ○
Vegetables   ○ ○ ○ ○
Calcium-Rich   ○ ○ ○
Protein-Rich   ○ ○ ○ ○
Breads/Grains   ○ ○ ○ ○ ○ ○ ○ ○ ○
Water   ○ ○ ○ ○ ○ ○ ○ ○

Fitness Tip

If you clench the railings of a stairclimber or treadmill, you'll burn far fewer calories than if you pump your arms. Don't exercise at such a high level that you're forced to grab on to the railings. It's okay, however, to grasp them lightly for balance.

Week 10 THURSDAY DATE

CARDIO EXERCISE | TIME | CALORIES BURNED

STRETCHING Yes [ ] No [ ]

NUTRITION Fat Budget _____

	Fat Grams	Low-Sugar Carb
Breakfast:		
Snack:		
Lunch:		
Snack:		
Dinner:		
Notes: **Totals:**		

FOOD GROUP SERVINGS

Fruits ○ ○ ○ ○ ○
Vegetables ○ ○ ○ ○
Calcium-Rich ○ ○ ○
Protein-Rich ○ ○ ○ ○
Breads/Grains ○ ○ ○ ○ ○ ○ ○ ○ ○
Water ○ ○ ○ ○ ○ ○ ○ ○

Food Fact

Brown sugar and raw sugar are no better than white sugar. Honey has minute amounts of a few minerals, but not enough to make a difference. It would take 11 cups of honey to meet your daily need for iron!

Week 10 FRIDAY

DATE

CARDIO EXERCISE

TIME

CALORIES BURNED

STRETCHING YES NO

NUTRITION FAT BUDGET _____

	FAT GRAMS	LOW-SUGAR CARB
Breakfast:		
Snack:		
Lunch:		
Snack:		
Dinner:		
Notes: **Totals:**		

FOOD GROUP SERVINGS

Fruits ○○○○○
Vegetables ○○○○
Calcium-Rich ○○○
Protein-Rich ○○○○
Breads/Grains ○○○○○○○○○○
Water ○○○○○○○○

Fitness Tip

During any given workout you can increase the number of calories you burn in two ways: by exercising longer or by exercising harder. Don't try to exercise longer and harder in the same workout! Walk 40 minutes instead of 30, or walk for 30 minutes at an 18-minute pace rather than a 20-minute pace.

Week 10 SATURDAY DATE

CARDIO EXERCISE | TIME | CALORIES BURNED

STRETCHING YES ☐ NO ☐

NUTRITION FAT BUDGET _____

	FAT GRAMS	LOW-SUGAR CARB
Breakfast:		
Snack:		
Lunch:		
Snack:		
Dinner:		
Notes: **Totals:**		

FOOD GROUP SERVINGS
Fruits ○○○○○
Vegetables ○○○○
Calcium-Rich ○○○
Protein-Rich ○○○○
Breads/Grains ○○○○○○○○○
Water ○○○○○○○○

Food Fact
Manufacturers introduced sugar-coated cereals in the 1940s to boost business. The gimmick worked—too well. Many cereals now contain sugar as the leading ingredient.

Week 10 SUNDAY DATE

CARDIO EXERCISE   TIME   CALORIES BURNED

STRETCHING YES   NO

NUTRITION FAT BUDGET _____

	FAT GRAMS	LOW-SUGAR CARB
Breakfast:		
Snack:		
Lunch:		
Snack:		
Dinner:		
Notes: **Totals:**		

FOOD GROUP SERVINGS

Fruits ○○○○○○

Vegetables ○○○○

Calcium-Rich ○○○

Protein-Rich ○○○○

Breads/Grains ○○○○○○○○○

Water ○○○○○○○○

Food Fact

Studies show that drinks with aspartame have no effect on curbing appetite, and they might actually trigger hunger, although the research is only preliminary.

WEEK IN REVIEW

TONING

DAYS [   ]   DID YOU MEET THE GOAL? _____

NOTES _____

_____

CARDIO EXERCISE

DAYS [   ]   CALORIES [   ]   DID YOU MEET THE GOALS? _____

NOTES _____

_____

WEIGHT [   ]

NUTRITION

DAYS UNDER FAT BUDGET [   ]   FOOD FOCUS RATING, 1–5 [   ]

you did it !
you should feel extremely
proud of yourself for sticking with
your log. Just remember :
Living healthy is a lifelong
process !
Kathy

Part III

The Stretches

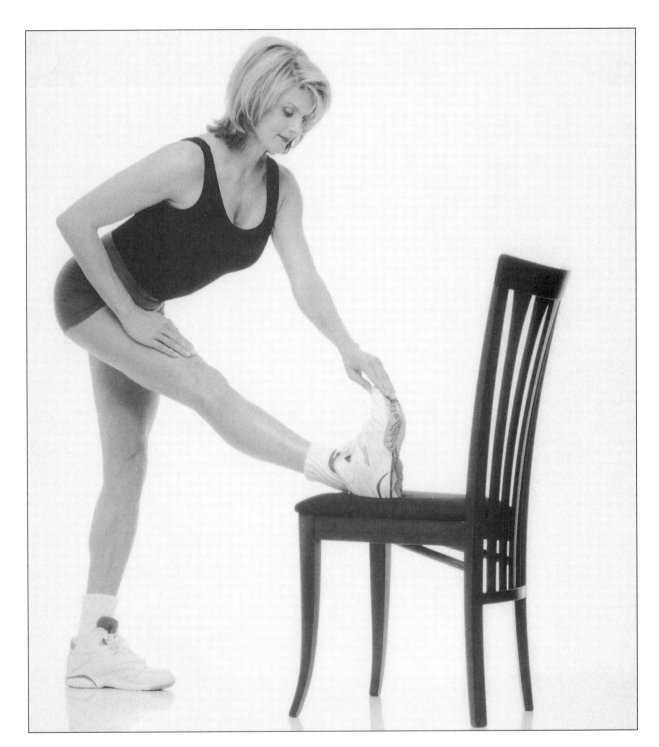

1. Back of the Thigh (Hamstring) and Calf

The Stretch: Raise your right leg and rest your foot on a chair seat. With your right leg straight and left knee slightly bent, lean forward from your hips, not your waist, and pull your toes back toward you. Repeat with your left leg extended.

The Focus: You shouldn't have to tilt your upper body very far forward before you feel the stretch in the back of your leg and your calf muscles.

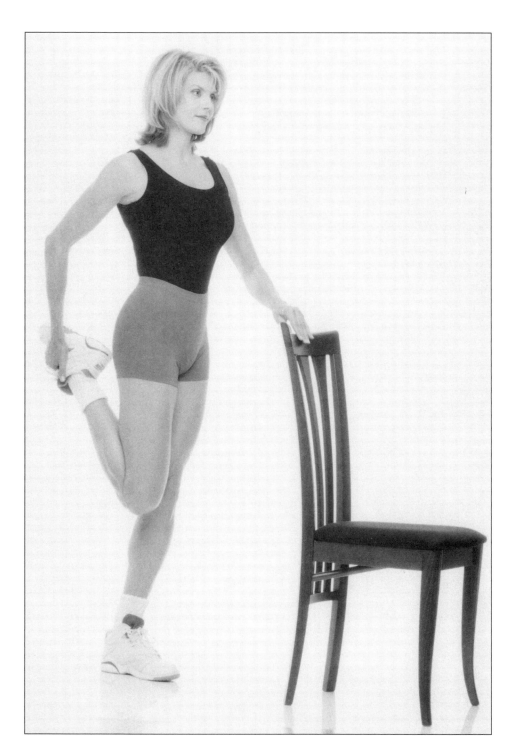

2. Front of the Thigh (Quadriceps), Hip Flexor, and Shin

The Stretch: Place your left hand on a chair for balance, and grasp your right foot behind you with your right hand. Pull your heel gently toward your buttocks. Keep your knees together and hips facing forward. Repeat with the other leg.

The Focus: By squeezing your buttocks and tucking them under slightly, you'll feel an even better stretch in the front of your thigh and hip. If you point your toe, you'll feel more of a stretch in the shin.

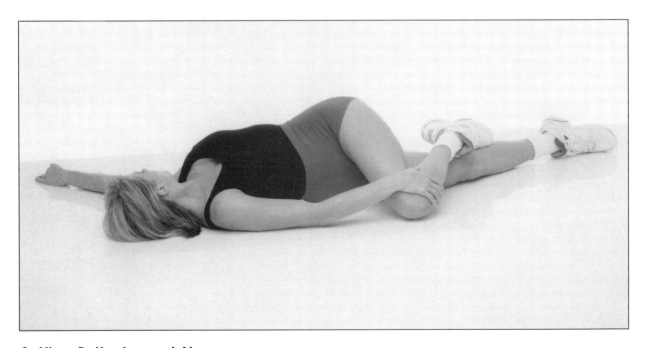

3. Hips, Buttocks, and Abs

The Stretch: Lying on your back, use your right hand to pull your left knee across your body and toward the ground on your right side. Keep your left shoulder flat on the ground with your arm outstretched. Repeat on the other side.

The Focus: By slightly altering where you place your bent leg, you'll feel the stretch in different parts of your hips and buttocks. Try moving your knee toward your head, then away from it. At first you may not be able to keep your shoulder flat on the floor, but you'll still get a good stretch in your abdominals.

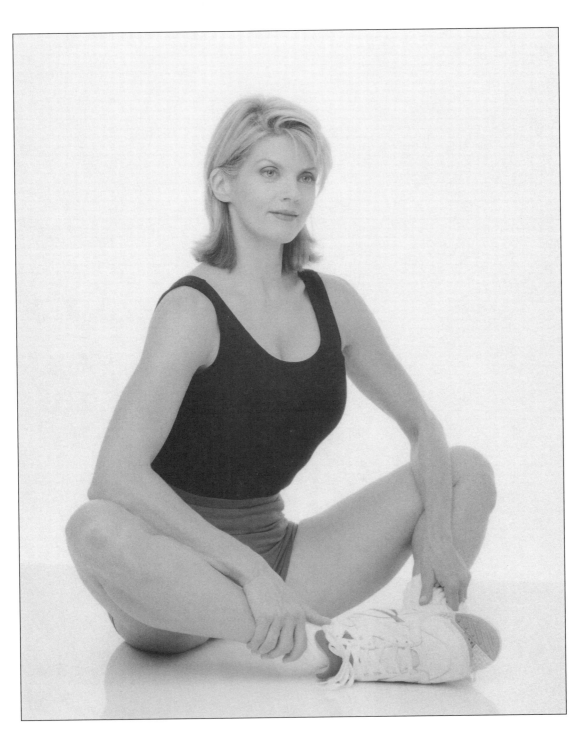

4. Inner Thigh (Adductors)

The Stretch: Sit on the floor and bring the soles of your feet together. Now bring your feet in as close to your buttocks as you comfortably can. Use your elbows to push your knees toward the floor.

The Focus: You should feel the stretch on the inside of your thighs. Lean forward from your hips. Try not to round your back as you push your knees toward the floor.

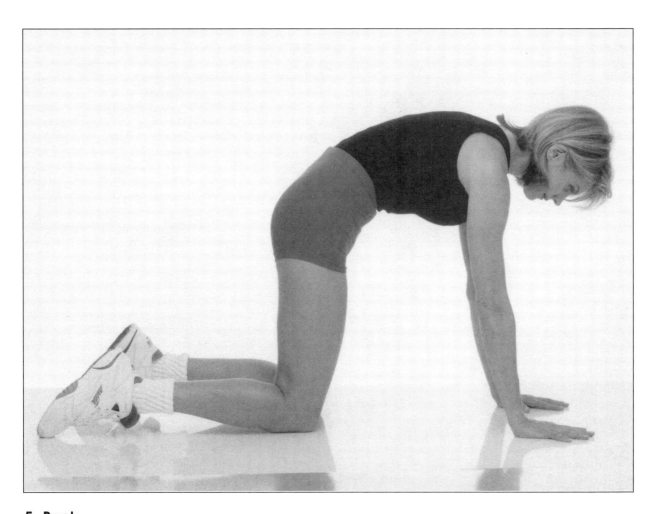

5. Back

The Stretch: Kneel on all fours with your hands and knees spread evenly and your neck relaxed. Tighten your abdominals, drop your head, and round your back up like a cat would. Hold, then return to starting position.

The Focus: By tightening your abdominal muscles—as if you're pulling your navel to the ceiling—you'll allow your back muscles to really relax and lengthen.

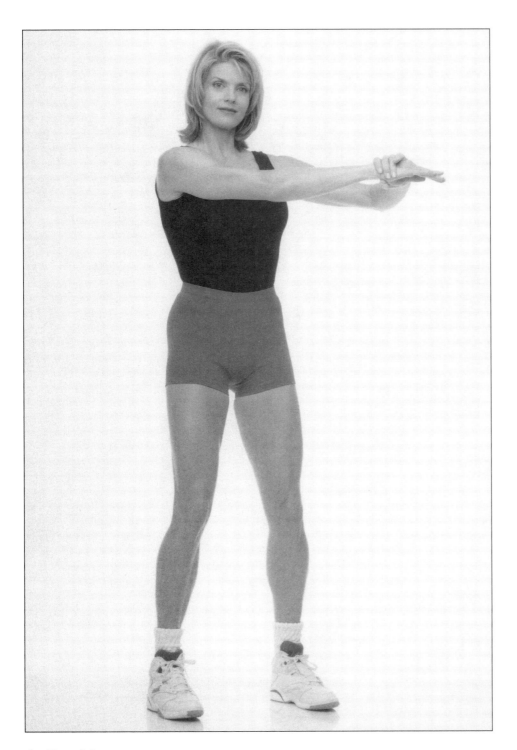

6. Shoulders

The Stretch: Stand with your knees slightly bent, and raise your right arm in front of you to shoulder height. Grasp your right arm with your left hand, and pull your right arm across your body. Repeat with your left arm.

The Focus: By moving your shoulder up toward your ears and then down as far as you can, you'll feel the stretch in slightly different areas of your shoulder and upper arm.

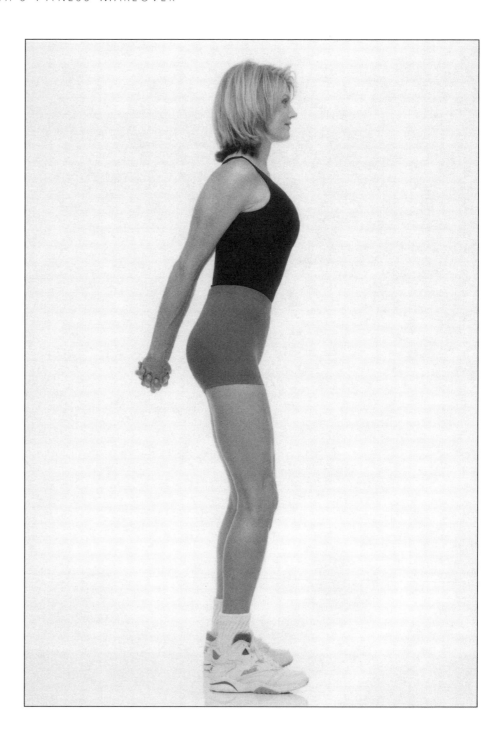

7. Chest

The Stretch: Stand with your feet hip-width apart and knees slightly bent. Clasp your hands behind your back. Straighten your arms, then lift your hands and chest.

The Focus: With your arms behind your back, take a deep breath and feel your chest expanding. You'll feel a stretch in the front of your shoulders, too.

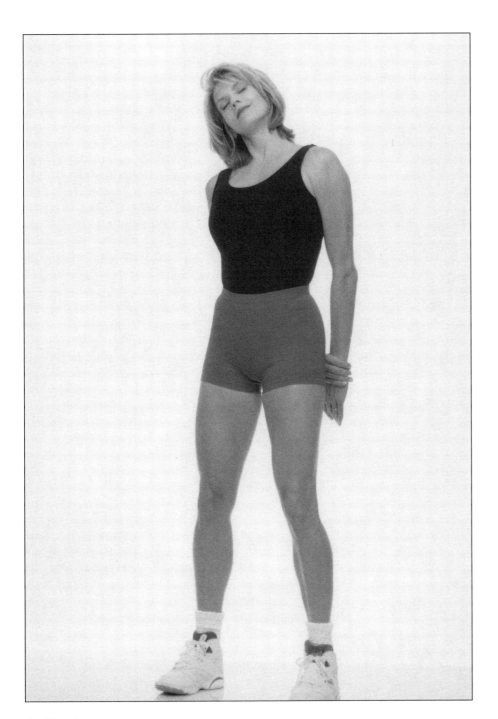

8. Neck

The Stretch: Stand with your feet hip-width apart and knees slightly bent. Drop your head forward, stretching the muscles in the back of your neck. Slowly lift your neck back up. Now place your hands behind your back, and grab your left wrist with your right hand. Drop your head to your right shoulder, and at the same time pull down on your left arm, stretching your neck and upper back. Bring your head back up, then repeat to the other side.

The Focus: As you hold the stretches, exhale and feel the release in the muscles that get tense from everyday activity. Perform these stretches gently.

Part IV

The Exercises

1. Crunch

Targets your abdominal muscles.

The Setup: Lie on your back with your knees bent and feet flat on the floor. Place your hands behind your head, and keep your neck relaxed; don't push your chin up or pull it down into your chest. Keep your elbows comfortably out to the side.

The Move: Exhale, tighten your abdominals, and pull your rib cage toward your hips, lifting your head, neck, and shoulder blades off the ground as one unit. Remember: This isn't an old-fashioned sit-up—you don't need to lift more than a couple of inches off the floor. Pause at the top of the movement, then inhale as you slowly lower all the way back down.

The Focus: Concentrate on pulling your rib cage down, as opposed to lifting your head and shoulders up. Make sure the movement comes from your abs—not your neck or shoulders. Use your hands only to *support* your head, not lift it.

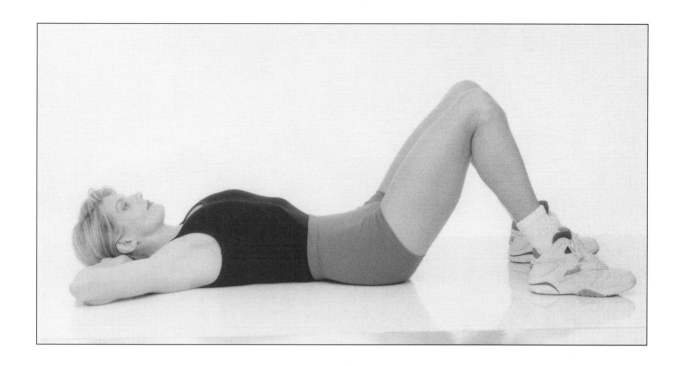

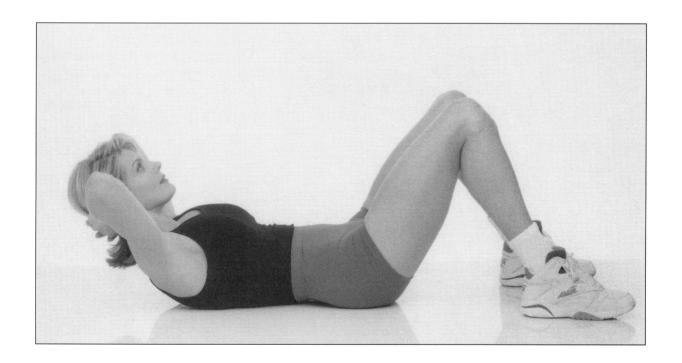

2. Reverse Curl

Targets the lower portion of your abdominal muscles.

The Setup: Lie on your back with your knees lined up directly over your hips. Your heels should hang down near the back of your thighs. Rest your arms on the floor beside you at a 45-degree angle from your body, palms facing down.

The Move: Exhale, tighten your abdominals, and tilt your hips off the floor. Pause at the top of the move, inhale, and lower back down. This is a subtle move—your hips barely need to clear the floor.

The Focus: Concentrate on lifting with the lower part of your abdominal muscles, *not* your front hip muscles. Don't kick or swing your legs. Try not to push on the floor with your hands; if you're tempted, place your hands behind your head.

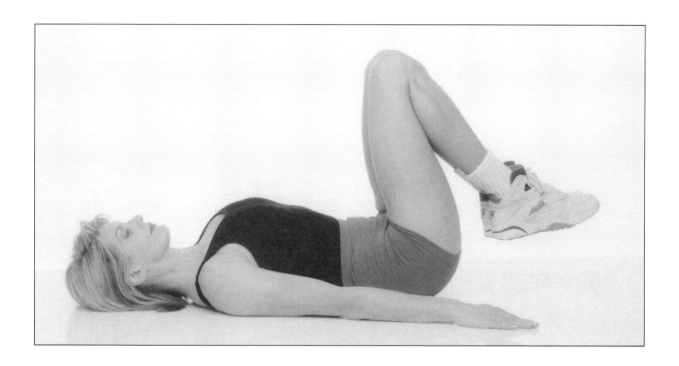

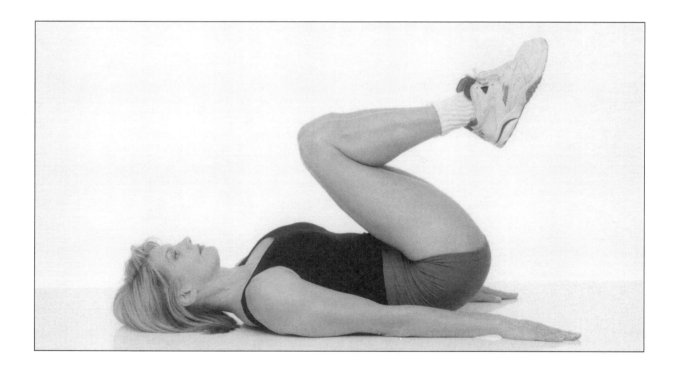

3. Cross Crunch

Targets your waist and abdominal muscles.

The Setup: Lie on your back with your knees bent and feet flat on the floor. Place your hands behind your head, elbows comfortably out to the side, and keep your neck relaxed, as in the Crunch.

The Move: Exhale. As you curl your head, neck, and shoulder blades off the floor, rotate your torso, pulling the left side of your rib cage toward your right inner thigh. Pause at the top, inhale, and slowly lower back down. You can do all of your repetitions on one side before switching sides, or you can alternate sides throughout each set. Be sure to do the recommended number of repetitions *for each side*.

The Focus: Make sure you rotate only your torso—not your arms and neck. Keep your elbows in line with your ears throughout the movement. Concentrate on pulling your rib cage down and across rather than pulling your elbows across.

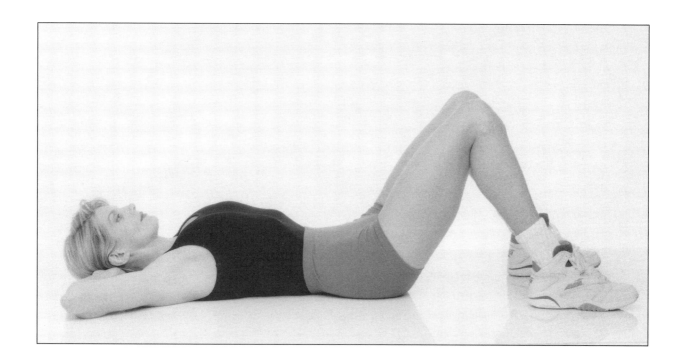

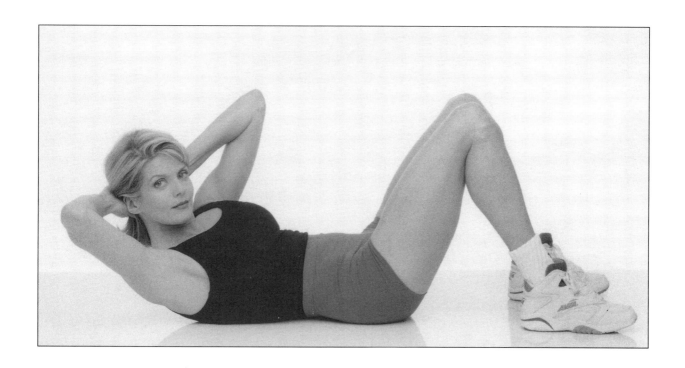

4. Back Extension

Targets your lower back muscles.

The Setup: Lie on your stomach with your feet down and forehead resting on your hands, elbows out to the side.

The Move: Keeping your neck straight, exhale, and slowly lift your chest off the floor using your lower back muscles. Pause at the top, inhale, and lower back to starting position. Keep the tops of your feet on the floor—don't kick your legs up into a "Superman" position! That can place excess stress on your lower back.

The Focus: Don't lift your head; concentrate on using those back muscles to raise your torso. Keep your eyes focused on the floor and your elbows out to the side. Lift only as high as you comfortably can—an inch or two is fine.

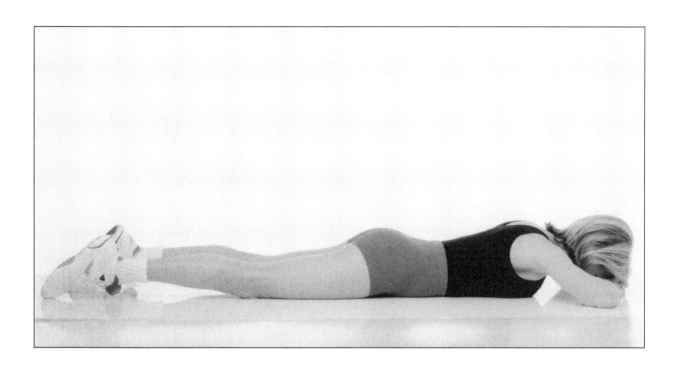

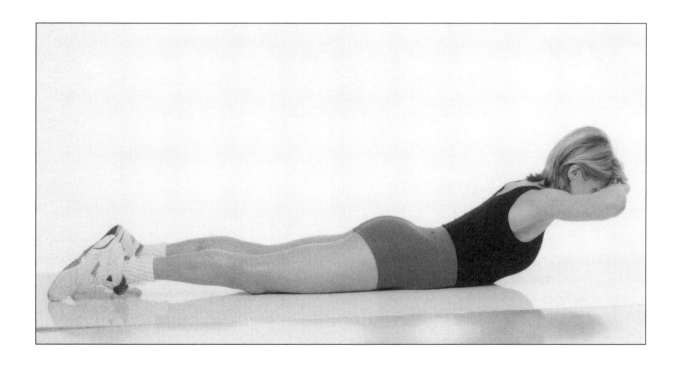

5. Back Extension with a Twist

Targets your lower back muscles.

The Setup: As in the Back Extension, lie on your stomach with your feet down, forehead resting on your hands, and elbows out to the sides.

The Move: This is a four-count movement: 1) Exhale, and lift your chest off the floor. 2) Twist your torso to the left until your right elbow touches the floor and your left elbow points diagonally toward the ceiling. 3) Return to center. 4) Inhale, and lower back down. Alternate sides until you've completed the recommended number of repetitions for *each* side.

The Focus: Let your lower back muscles do all the work. As you twist from your torso, don't rotate your neck; just let your head go along for the ride naturally. Don't let your feet lift off the ground.

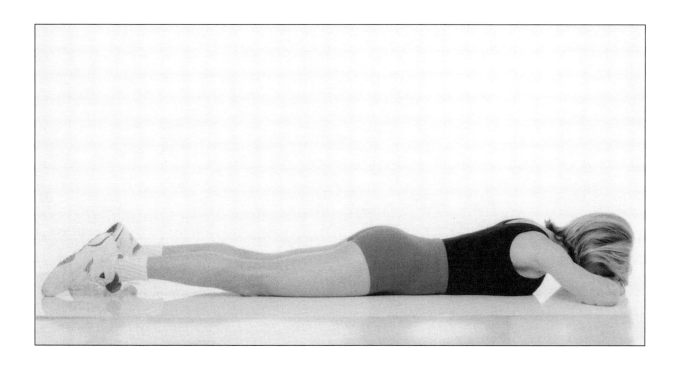

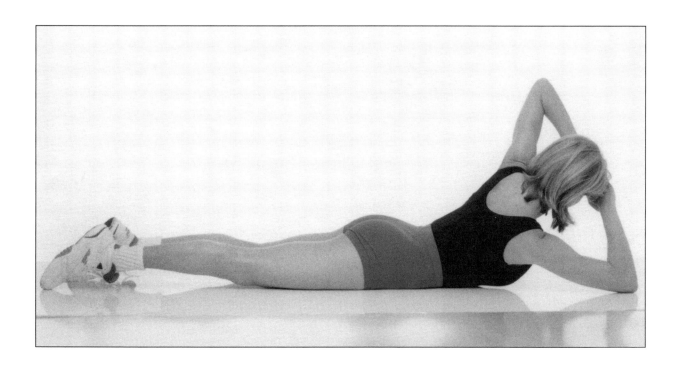

6. Hip Lift

Targets the buttocks and back of thighs.

The Setup: Lie on your back on the floor with your heels resting on the seat of a chair and legs straight. Rest your arms on the floor slightly away from your body.

The Move: Exhale. Press your heels into the chair, squeeze your buttocks muscles, and lift your body up until it's in a straight line from your shoulders to your heels. Pause, inhale, and slowly lower back down.

The Focus: Lift at a slow, controlled speed instead of throwing your body up in the air. Keep your back straight, not arched. Make sure you feel the weight across your shoulders, not on your head or the back of your neck.

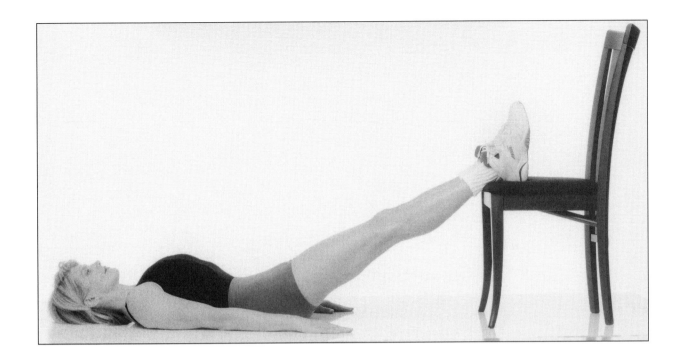

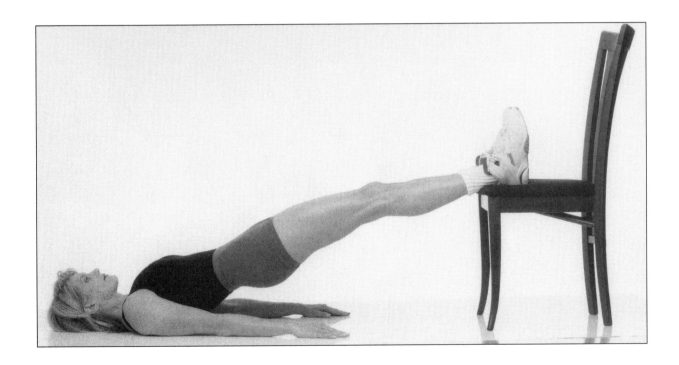

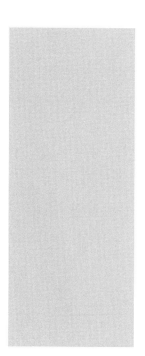

7. Backward Lunge

Targets your buttocks plus back and front of thighs.

The Setup: Stand up straight with your abdominals tightened, arms hanging by your sides, and feet slightly apart.

The Move: Inhale, and take a large step back with your right leg, keeping your arms by your sides. Bend both knees so your left knee is directly over your left ankle and your right knee points to the floor with your heel lifted. Your left thigh should be parallel to the floor. Exhale, and push off your right toes back to starting position. Alternate legs, doing the recommended number of repetitions for each leg.

The Focus: Throughout each repetition, keep slightly more weight on your front leg. If you have trouble balancing, place a chair at your side and grasp it lightly with one hand. When this exercise becomes easy, hold a dumbbell in each hand.

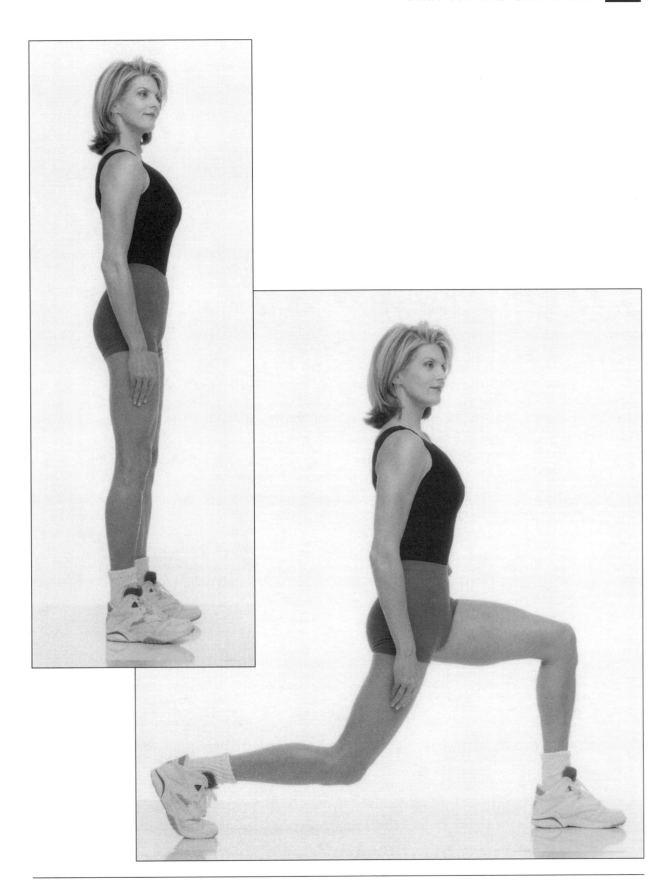

8. Leg Lift
(Ankle weights optional.)

Targets your buttocks and back of thigh.

The Setup: Stand a foot or two away from the back of a chair. Lean forward and rest your elbows on the chair. Move your right leg slightly behind your left so that your right toes are on the floor near your left heel. Your right heel is off the ground.

The Move: Exhale, and slowly lift your right leg as high as you can without arching your back. Pause, inhale, and lower back down.

The Focus: As you lean forward, bend from the hip—don't round your back. When you lift, your knee and toe may turn slightly to the outside. This is natural.

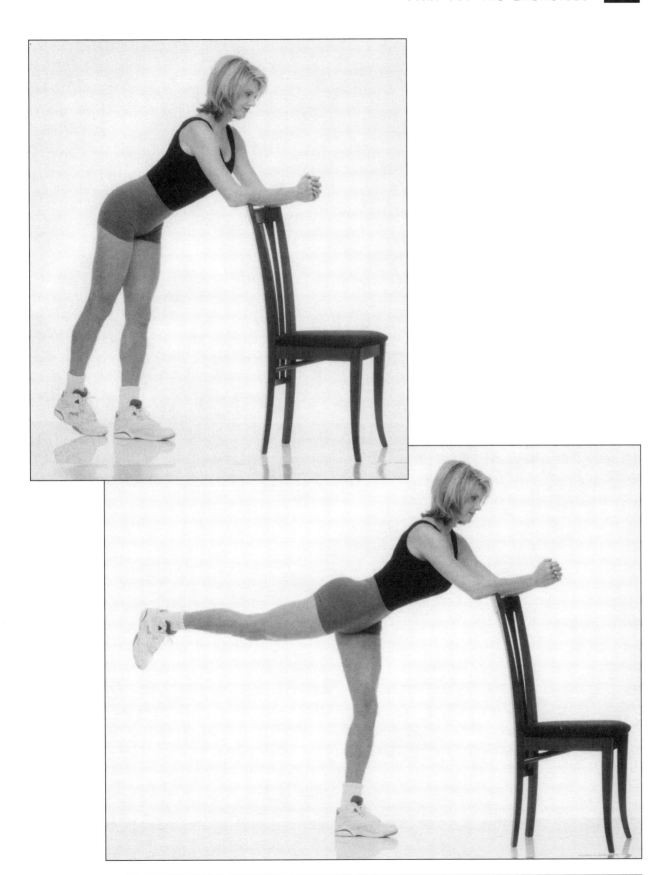

9. Squat

Targets the front and rear thigh muscles and buttocks.

The Setup: Stand up straight with your abdominals tightened, feet hip-width apart and hands by your sides.

The Move: Inhale, bend your knees as if you're going to sit in a chair, and lower down until your thighs are nearly parallel to the floor. Meanwhile, lift your arms out in front of you for balance. Pause, exhale, and slowly stand up.

The Focus: As you lower down, make sure your tailbone points back. Keep your chest lifted and back straight, not rounded. Finally, don't let your knees shoot out past your toes. When this exercise gets easy, hold dumbbells by your sides.

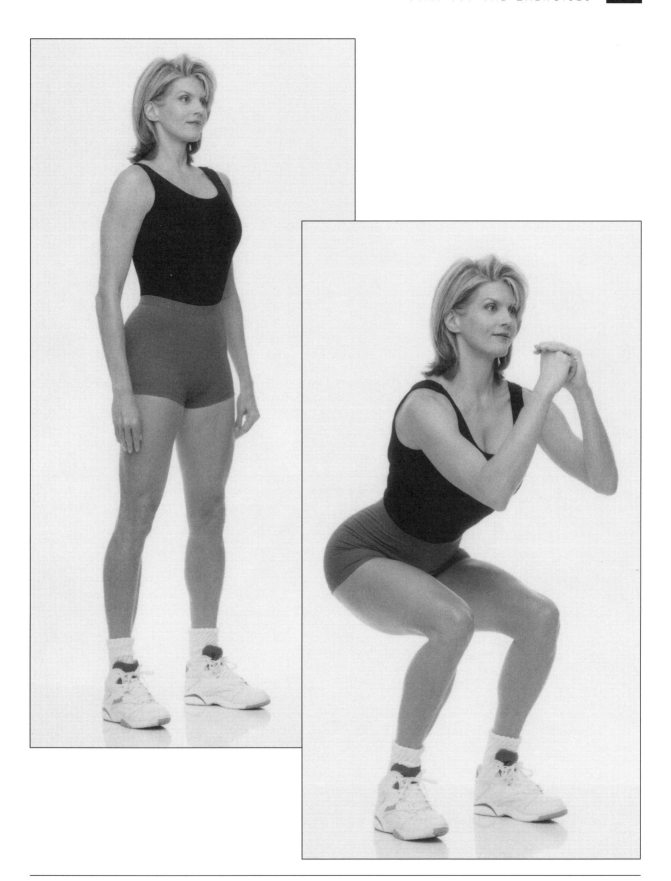

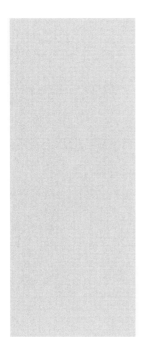

10. Standing Side Lift
(Ankle weights optional.)

Targets your outer hip muscles.

The Setup: Stand up straight with your abdominals tightened and your left side facing the back of a chair. Lean slightly to the side, resting your left elbow on the chair. Bring your right arm across your body, placing your hand on the top of the chair for balance.

The Move: Exhale, and slowly lift your right leg out to the side, keeping your knee and foot facing forward. Lift as high as you can without turning your knee and toe up to the ceiling. Pause at the top, inhale, and lower back down.

The Focus: Make sure your leg is lifting directly out to the side, not behind you. Your supporting leg muscles are working to keep you balanced and upright.

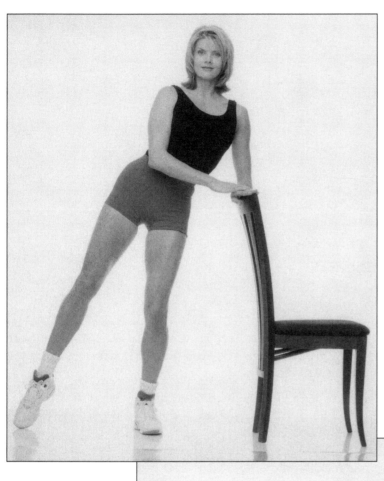

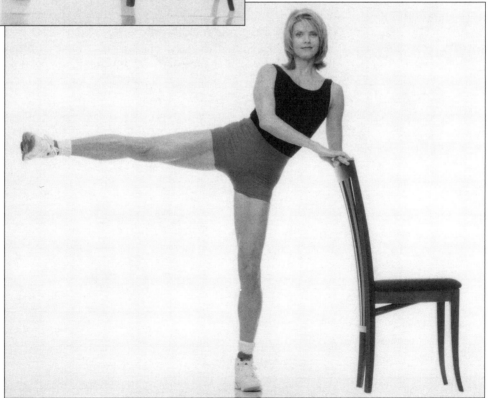

11. Inner Thigh Pull

Targets your inner thigh muscles.

The Setup: Stand with your feet wide enough apart to feel a slight stretch in your inner thighs. Bend your knees, turn your toes out slightly, tighten your abdominals, and place your hands on your hips.

The Move: Exhale, and drag your right foot toward your left foot, using the floor as resistance. Keep dragging until your feet are together and legs are straight, with your toes turned out slightly (like "first position" in ballet). Inhale, take a wide step to the side with your *left* foot, then drag it in. Continue alternating legs.

The Focus: Drag your foot enough so that you really feel your inner thigh muscles working. Imagine that you have one foot on a dock and the other foot on a boat three feet away, and you're trying to pull the boat in to the dock. Keep the sole of your foot flat on the floor; don't drag the inside of your shoe.

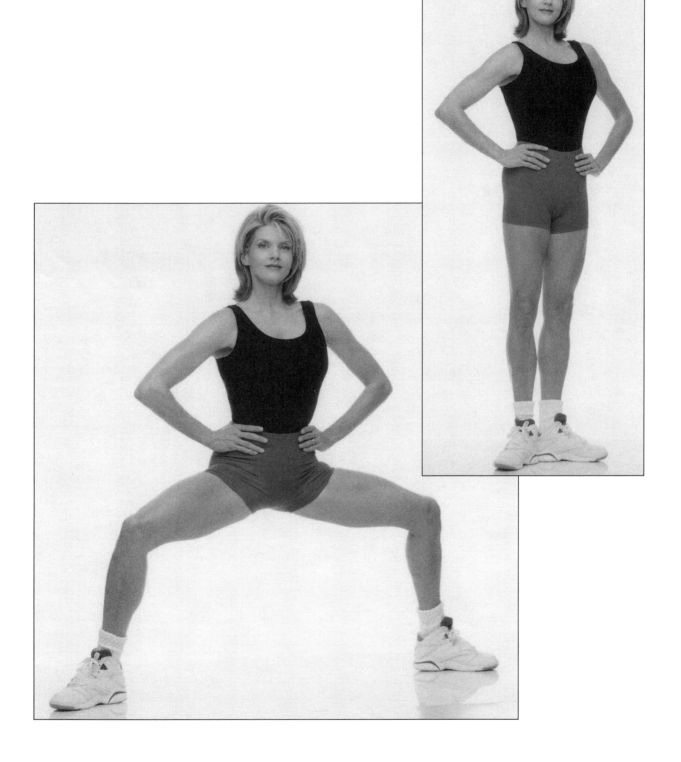

12. Hamstring Curl

Targets rear thigh muscles and buttocks.

The Setup: Lie on your back with your knees bent and heels on the seat of a chair. Your lower legs should be parallel to the ground, thighs perpendicular. Place your arms on the floor out to the side for balance.

The Move: Exhale, and press your heels down into the chair as if you were pulling them toward the back of your thighs. Keep pushing them down until your hips lift off the floor. Pause at the top, inhale, and slowly lower back down.

The Focus: Make your hamstrings do the work. Rather than use your buttocks to push your hips up, lift your hips by really squeezing your heels down.

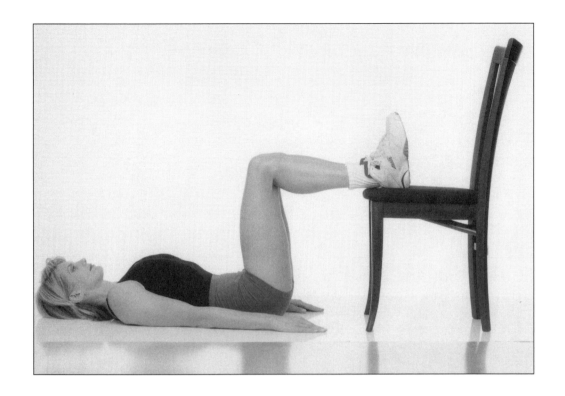

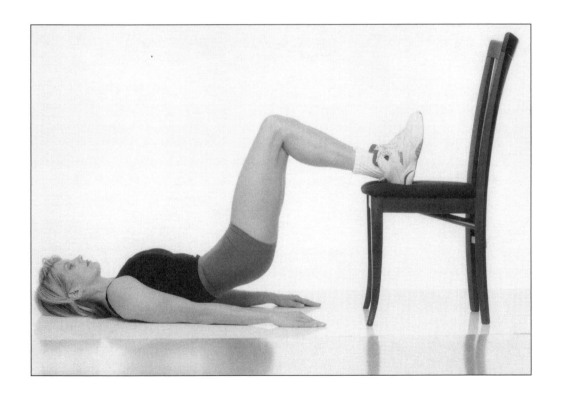

13. One-Arm Row

(Use your medium or heavy dumbbell.)

Targets your middle back, upper back, rear of shoulder, and front of upper arm.

The Setup: Stand with your right foot on the floor and left knee resting on a chair seat. Lean forward and place your left hand on the seat in front of your left knee. Keep your back straight and parallel to the floor. Your right arm should hang straight down, dumbbell in hand.

The Move: Exhale, and bend your elbow, lifting the dumbbell until your elbow is higher than your back and the dumbbell is close to your underarm. Keep your palm facing your body. Pause at the top, inhale, and lower back down.

The Focus: Keep your palm facing in and your elbow pointing back—don't let it swing out to the side. Also, keep both shoulders facing the floor; don't let your body tip to the side.

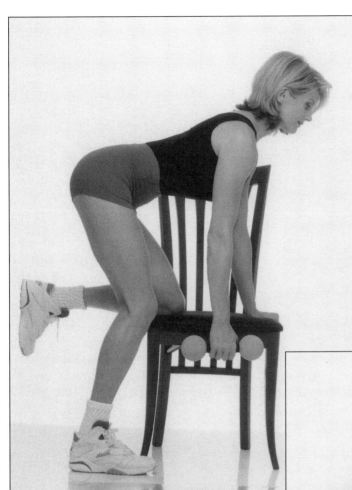

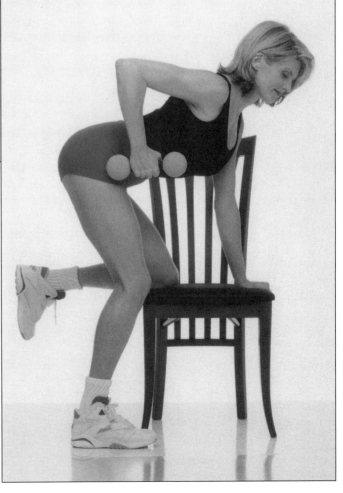

14. Seated Back Flye

(Use your lightest dumbbells.)

Targets the upper back and rear of shoulders.

The Setup: Sit on a chair with a pillow on your lap and lean forward, letting your chest rest on the pillow. Grasping your lightest dumbbells, let your arms hang down to the sides. (Practice this exercise a few times with no weight.)

The Move: Exhale, squeeze your shoulder blades together, and slowly lift your arms out to the side until they're slightly higher than shoulder level. Pause, inhale, and lower back down.

The Focus: Make sure your arms lift directly out to the side, not behind you. Keep your shoulder blades squeezed when you lift the weights *and* when you lower them. Release your shoulder blades at the bottom of the movement.

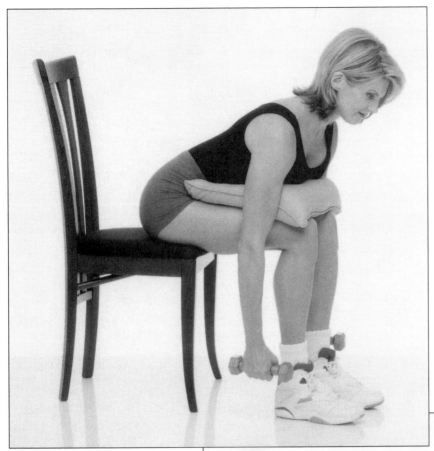

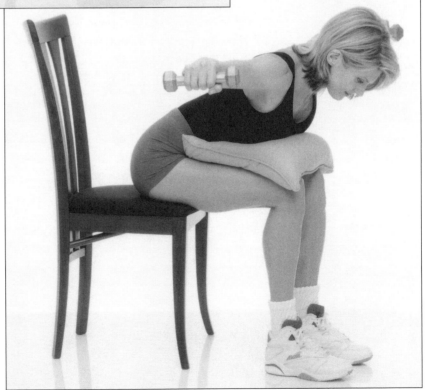

15. Push-up

Targets your chest, front of shoulders, and back of upper arm.

The Setup: Kneel on the ground with your arms lined up so that your wrists are directly beneath your shoulders and fingertips turned in slightly. Walk your hands forward until your body is at an angle from your knees up to your shoulders. Keep your neck straight.

The Move: Inhale, and bend your elbows, lowering your body down until your chest nears the floor. Pause, exhale, and press back up to starting position.

The Focus: Hold your abdominal muscles in tight so that your body is in a straight line as you lower it. Don't let your back sag as your arms get tired. Keep your shoulders over your wrists the whole time; avoid the tendency to push your weight back when you get tired. If you can't lower your body all the way down, start with a quarter push-up and gradually progress lower. When the kneeling push-up gets easy, straighten out your legs and balance on your toes.

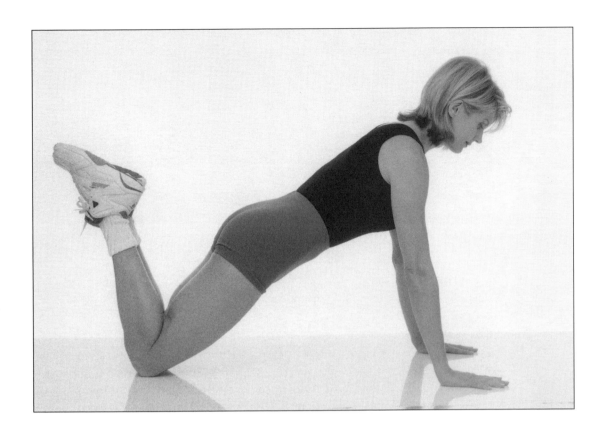

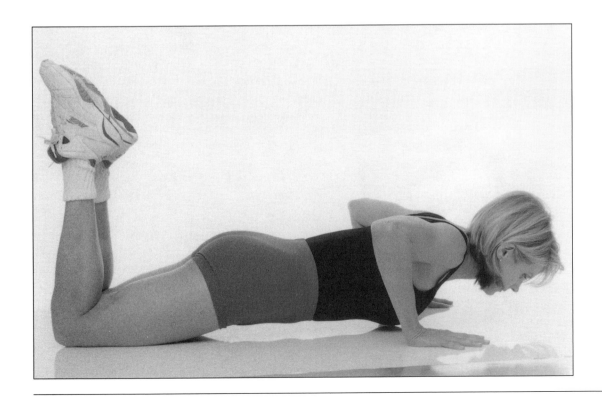

16. Chest Flye

(Use your medium or heavy dumbbells.)

Targets the chest and front shoulder muscles.

The Setup: Holding a dumbbell in each hand, lie on your back with a firm pillow under your head, shoulders, and upper back. Push your arms straight up until your elbows are almost straight and palms face each other. The dumbbells should be directly above your shoulders.

The Move: Inhale, then slowly lower your arms out to the sides, keeping your elbows slightly bent. Continue to lower until your elbows are slightly below your shoulders or you feel a gentle stretch in your chest and shoulder muscles. Pause, exhale, and slowly close your arms back up to starting position.

The Focus: Keep your wrists straight, almost as if you were wearing a cast on each one. In the starting position you should feel like you're hugging a big beach ball. As you lower your arms, imagine that the ball is getting bigger, pushing your arms open. To really target the chest, keep your arms in line with your shoulders; at the end of the movement, your body should look like a lower-case T.

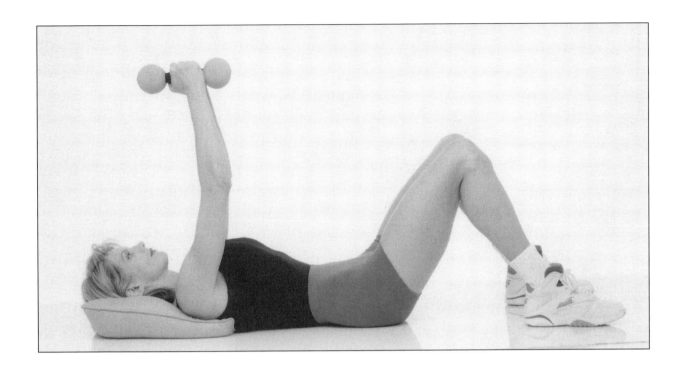

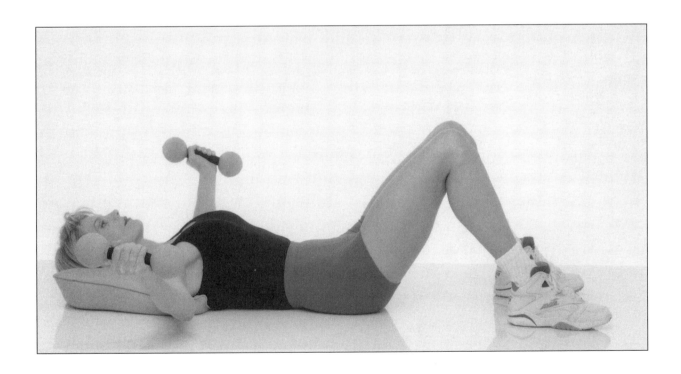

17. Lateral Raise
(Use your light or medium dumbbells.)

Targets the center shoulder muscles.

The Setup: Stand with your feet hip-width apart, knees slightly bent, abdominals tightened, and arms hanging by your sides. Hold a dumbbell in each hand, palms facing in.

The Move: Exhale, and slowly lift your arms out to the side until the dumbbells are slightly higher than your shoulders. Pause, inhale, and slowly lower back down.

The Focus: Lift directly out to the side; don't let the dumbbells end up in front of your thighs. At the top of the movement, let your thumbs turn slightly upward. Keep your elbows slightly bent, not locked.

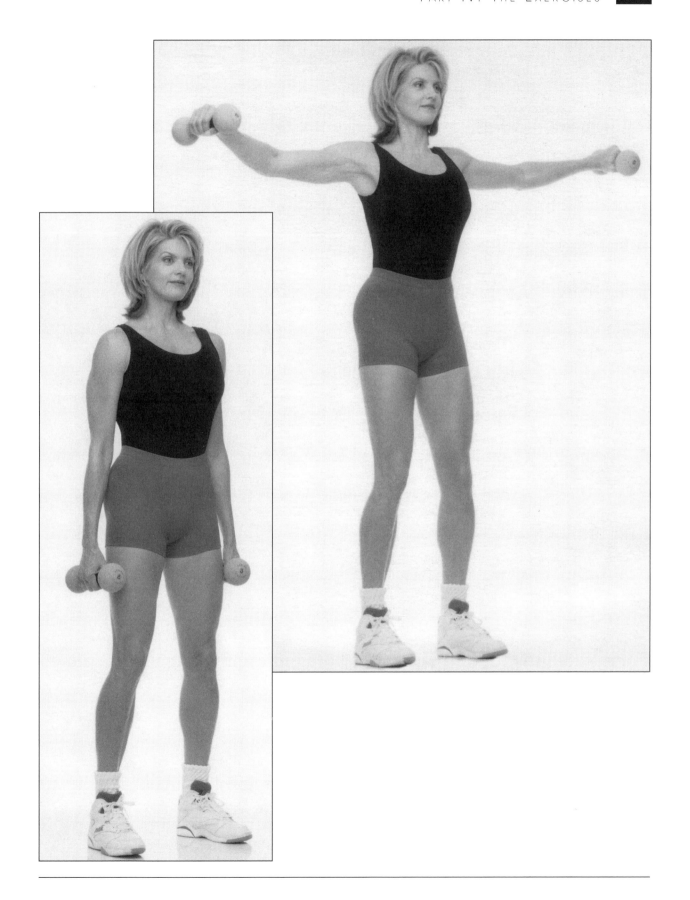

18. Front Raise

(Use your light or medium dumbbells.)

Targets the front shoulder muscles.

The Setup: Stand with your feet hip-width apart, knees slightly bent, abdominals tightened, and arms hanging by your sides. Hold a dumbbell in each hand, palms facing in.

The Move: Exhale, and slowly raise your arms in front of you until the dumbbells are slightly higher than your shoulders. Pause, inhale, and lower back down.

The Focus: Keep your elbows slightly bent, and don't allow your arms to lift higher than your shoulders. Keep your palms facing down the whole time. Try not to lean back as you lift, and don't swing the weights.

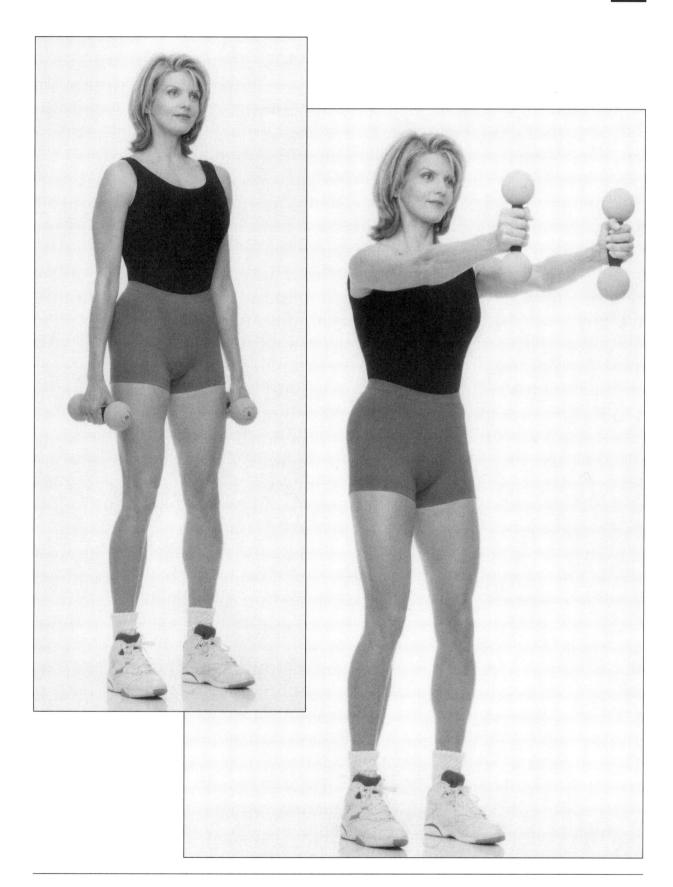

19. Rear Raise
(Use your light or medium dumbbells.)

Targets the rear shoulders and back of upper arm.

The Setup: Stand with your feet hip-width apart, knees slightly bent, abdominals tightened, and arms hanging by your sides. Hold a dumbbell in each hand, palms facing in.

The Move: Exhale, and lift your arms behind you as high as you can. Pause, exhale, and slowly lower back down. Keep your palms facing in.

The Focus: As you lift your arms back, try not to lean forward. Keep your body upright. Don't let your arms flare out to the side; lift them directly behind you.

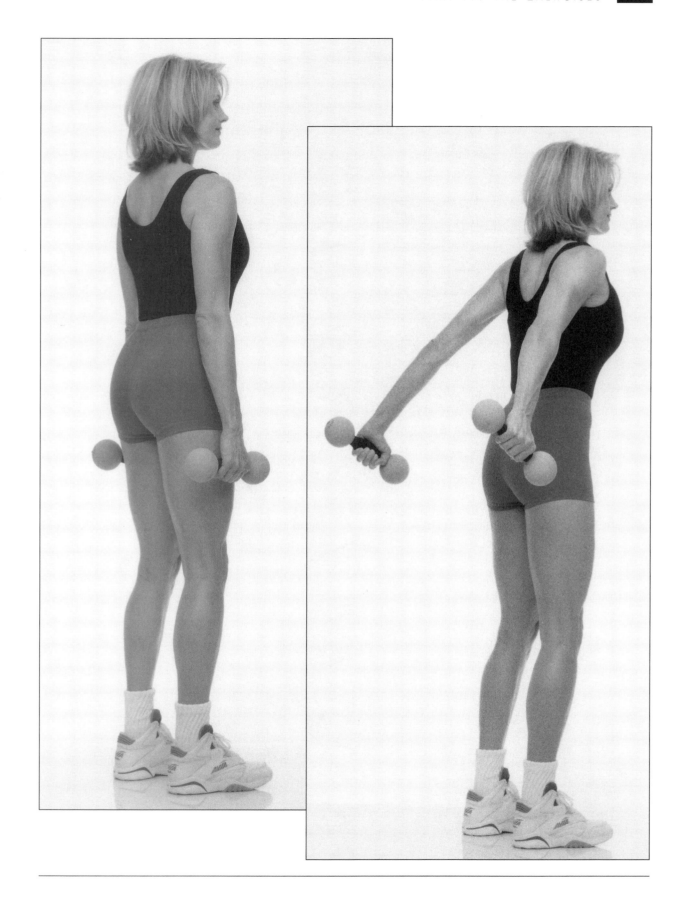

20. French Press
(Use your light or medium dumbbells.)

Targets the back of your upper arm.

The Setup: Lie on your back with a firm pillow underneath your head, shoulders, and upper back. Bend your knees and place your feet flat on the floor. Pick up the dumbbells and push them straight up in the air until your arms are straight, palms facing in.

The Move: Exhale, and slowly bend your elbows, lowering the dumbbells behind your head until they almost touch your shoulders. Pause at the bottom of the movement, inhale, and straighten your elbows.

The Focus: Concentrate on keeping your elbows pointed straight in the air throughout the entire movement. Don't let your arms move forward or back—you're not waving a flag back and forth!

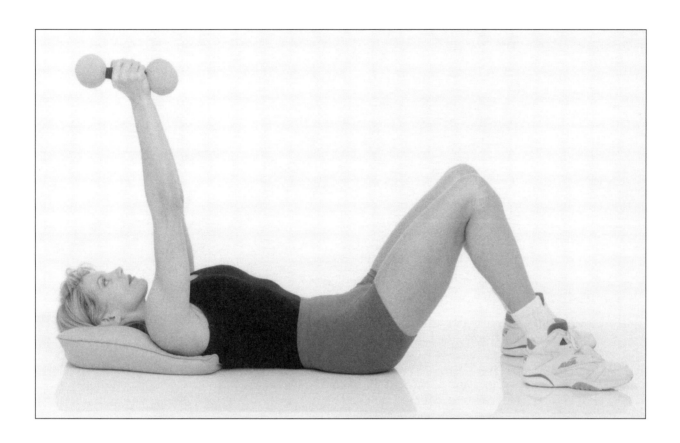

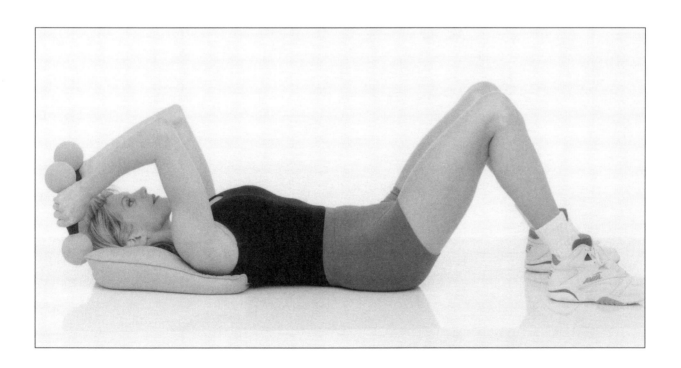

21. Triceps Kickback
(Use your light or medium dumbbells.)

Targets the back of your upper arm.

The Setup: Lean forward, place your left hand on the seat of a chair, and stagger your feet so your right leg is in front of your left and both knees are slightly bent. Holding a dumbbell in your right hand, lift your arm until your elbow is slightly higher than your body and the dumbbell points to the floor, palm facing in.

The Move: Exhale, then slowly straighten your elbow until your arm is straight. Pause at the top of the movement, inhale, and return to starting position.

The Focus: Throughout the exercise, keep your upper arm still, your back straight, and both shoulders facing the floor.

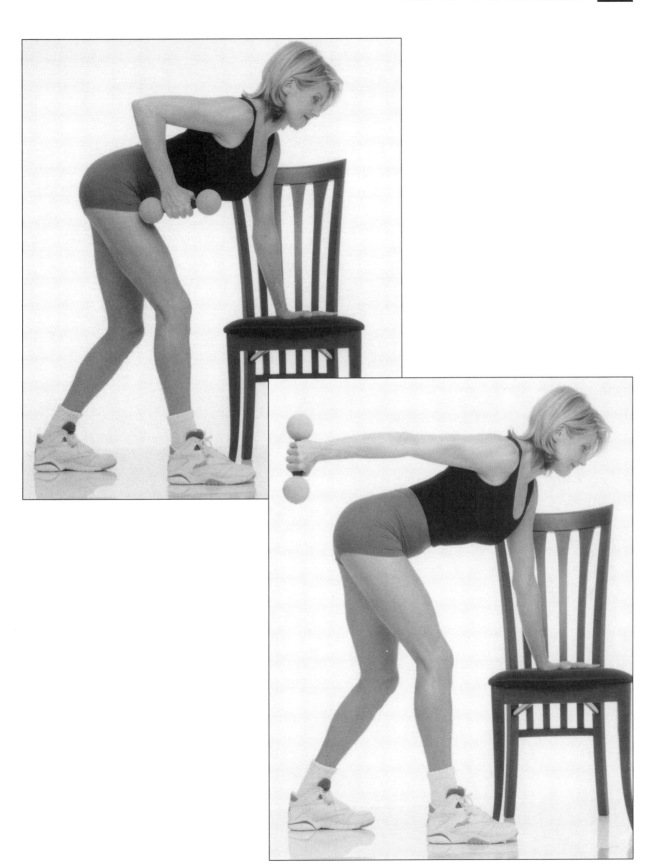

22. Seated Biceps Curl

(Use your medium dumbbells.)

Targets the front of your upper arm.

The Setup: Sit up straight in a chair with your feet flat on the floor. Hold a dumbbell in each hand with your arms hanging by your sides, palms facing in.

The Move: Exhale, and slowly bend your elbows, curling the dumbbells up to your shoulders. As you bend your elbows, gradually rotate your palms so that at the top of the movement they are facing your shoulders. Inhale, and slowly lower back down.

The Focus: As you curl the dumbbells, keep your elbows close to your sides. Don't swing your arms back and forth from the shoulder.

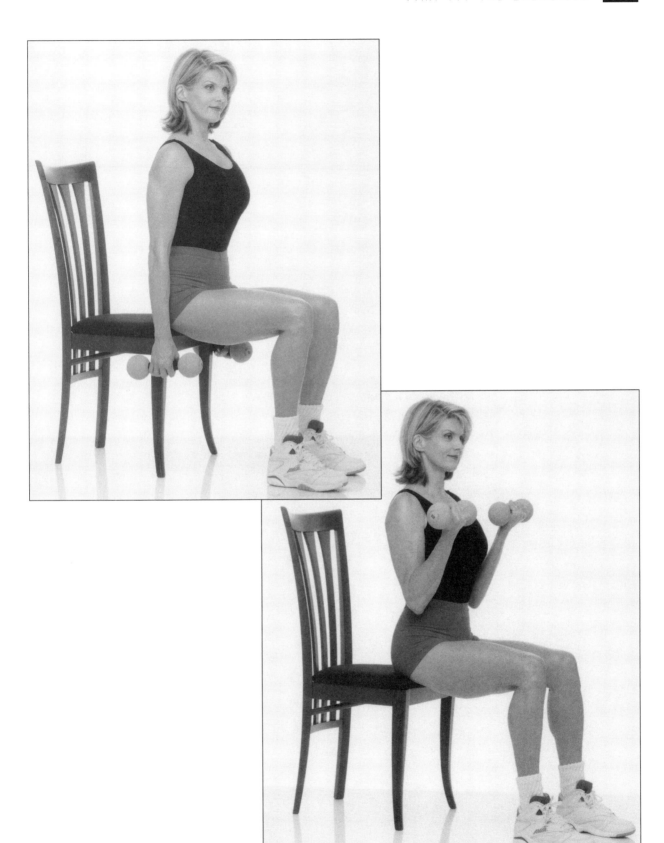

23. Concentration Curl

(Use a medium dumbbell.)

Targets the front of your upper arm.

The Setup: Sit on a chair, lean forward, and let your left palm rest on your left thigh. Holding a dumbbell in your right hand, rest the back of your right arm against the inside of your right thigh. Your right palm should face your left ankle.

The Move: Exhale, slowly bend your right elbow, and gradually rotate your palm so it faces your shoulder at the top of the movement.

The Focus: Curl the weight as high as you can, squeezing your biceps at the top of the move. Lift and lower the weight at the same speed.

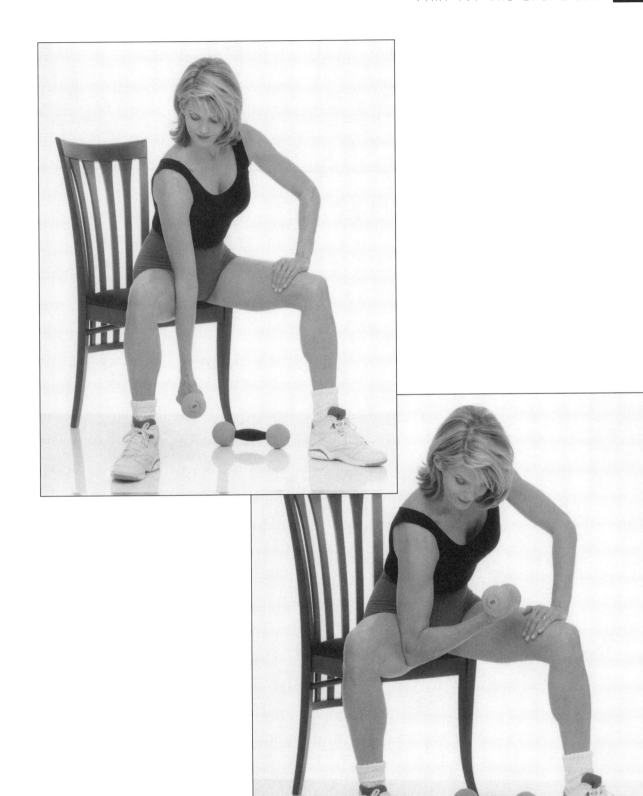

24. Standing Calf Raise

Targets your calf muscles.

The Setup: Stand on a sturdy platform facing the back of the chair, and rest both hands on the seat back for balance. Balance on the balls of your feet with your heels hanging off the edge of the platform.

The Move: Inhale, and slowly lower your heels until you feel a gentle stretch in your calf muscles. Exhale, and push up onto the balls of your feet, lifting your heels as high as you can. Pause at the top, inhale, and lower back down.

The Focus: As you lift up, keep equal weight across all 10 toes. Counteract the tendency to roll your feet outward by pressing the big-toe side of your foot into the floor. To keep your balance, pull your abdominal muscles in and keep your buttocks tucked. Lift and lower at the same speed, taking two slow counts in each direction.

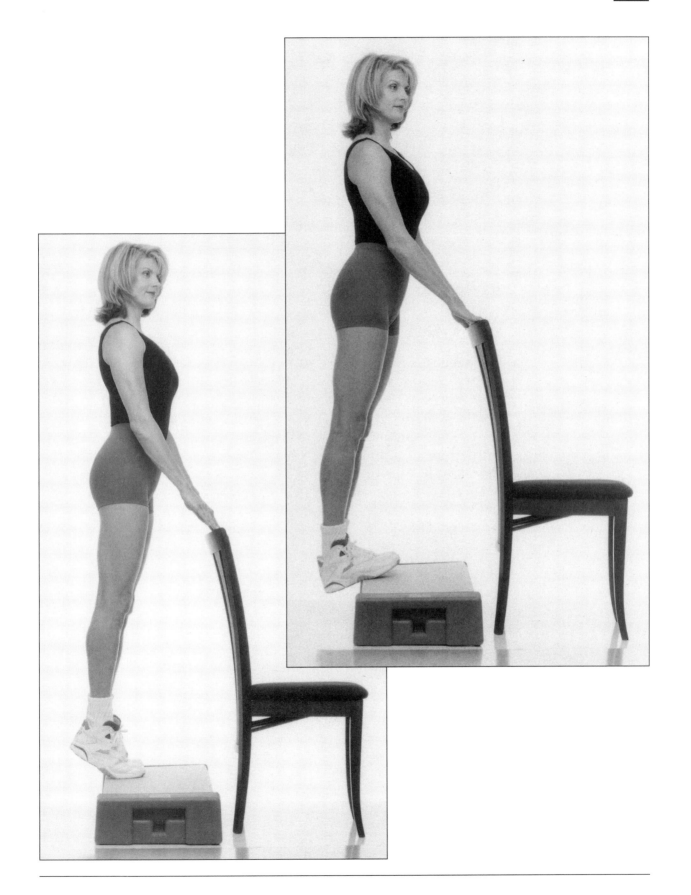

25. Toe Raise

Targets your shin muscles.

The Setup: Sit up straight in a chair with your feet flat on the floor. Place your right heel on the top of your left foot near your toes. Place your hands on the sides of the chair seat to help keep your back straight.

The Move: Exhale, and lift the front of your left foot off the floor, gently pressing down with your right foot to create resistance. Pause at the top, inhale, and lower back down.

The Focus: Lift your toes as high as you can off the floor, but maintain good posture, making sure not to slump. Resist on the way up *and* on the way down, pushing gently with your right foot.

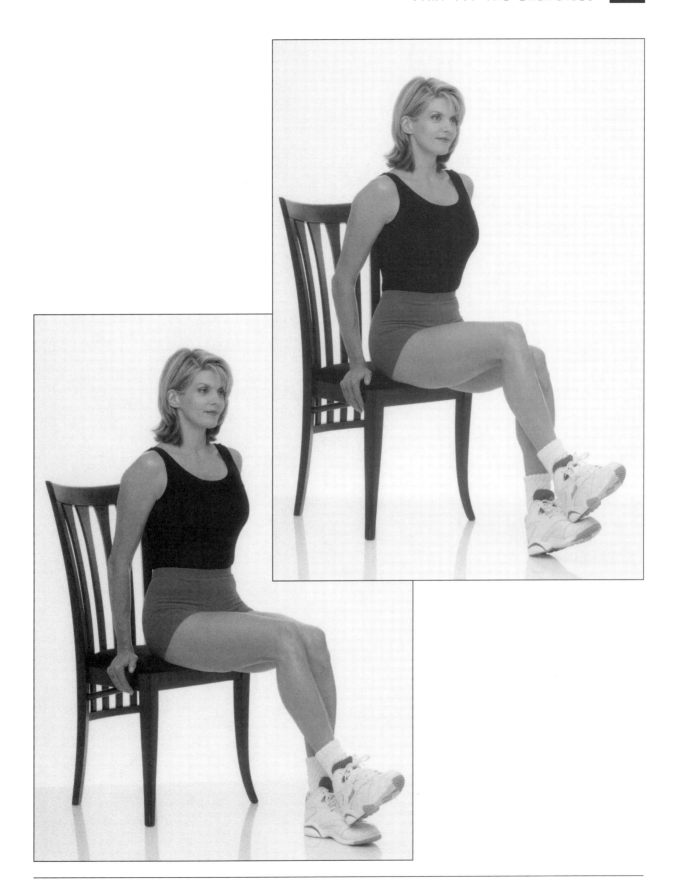

Index

Abdominal muscles, *vii,* 14, 23
    stretches, 203
    toning exercises, 210–11, 212–13, 214–15
abductors, 77
Abs. *See* Abdominal muscles
adductors, 14, 77, 203
Aerobic exercise, 4, 6
Americans
    amount of soda consumed, 190
    and high-sugar foods, 184
    new Four Food Groups, 58
    typical diet, 165–66
Amino acids, 93
Ankle weights, 4
Ankles, 185
Antioxidant nutrients, 166
Arms, 148–49, 166–67
    and shoulder muscles, 131
    See also Upper arm exercises
Arteries, 40
Aspartame, 184, 196
Avocados, 173

B vitamins, 173
Back. *See* Lower back; Upper back
Bagels, 69
Barley, 129
Beans, 76, 129, 130
Beta-carotene, 166
Biceps, 14, 148–49, 166–67
    See also Upper arm exercises
Bloating, 141
Blood pressure, 66, 176
Blood sugar levels, 76, 166
Body fat, 66
Bones, 112, 174
Brand Name Fat and Cholesterol Counter
    (American Heart Association), 8, 39
Bread
    white, 75
    whole grain, 75, 76, 88, 165–66
    whole wheat, 75, 76, 88, 183
Breakfast menus, 22
Breast cancer, 28
Butter, 41, 47
Buttocks
    discussed, 59
    plan for week, 60
    stretches, 202
    toning exercises, 220–21, 222–23, 224–25,
        226–27, 232–33

Calcium, *vii, ix,* 172
    best sources of, 112, 124
    daily minimums, 111, 118, 166
    discussed, 111–12
    plan for week, 114
    supplements, 121
Calories, 4, 31, 64, 65, 76, 82, 86, 93, 94,
    101
    burning of, 4, 12–13, 140
    discussed, 57–58
    plan for week, 60
    in sugar, 184–85

Calves, 185, 186
    stretch, 200
    toning exercise, 256–57
CamelBak, 148
Cancer, 28, 33, 129, 130, 131, 184
Carbohydrates, 83, 100, 157
    complex, 76, 94, 183
    discussed, 75–76
    plan for week, 78
Cardio Exercise Goals, 3–6, 12
Cardiovascular exercise, *viii–ix*
    benefits of, 176
    calories burned with, 12–13
    longer *vs.* harder workouts, 194
    for lower back pain, 41
    and moderation, 4–5, 192
    warm ups, 48
    and water, 147–48
    See also Cardio Exercise Goals; TONING
        EXERCISES
Center for Science and the Public Interest,
    51
Cereals, 195
CHARTS:
    Average Protein Content of Foods, 94
    Calcium Intake, 112
    Calorie Budget, 57
    Calories Burned, 12–13
    Complementary Proteins, 94
    Fiber Intake, 130
    Ideal Weight, 9
    Ideal Weight and Calories, 57
    Serving Sizes, 11
Chest muscles, 113
    toning exercises, 238–39, 240–41
Chips Ahoy cookies, 67
Cholesterol levels, 40, 46, 176
    and saturated fat, 39–40
    and soluble fibers, 130
Chromium, 166
Clinical depression, 191
Colds and flu, 176
Colon cancer, 129, 131
Complex carbohydrates, 76, 94, 183
Constipation, 130–31
Coronary artery disease, 49
Cottage cheese, 93
Cycling, 4, 140, 148

Daily Log. *See* Log
Dairy products, 111, 112, 124
Dannon Vanilla Yogurt, 184
Dehydration, 147–48, 154–55
Diabetes, 66, 176
Diarrhea, 141
Diet soda, *vii,* 184
Diets
    of Americans, 58, 165–66
    balanced, 7
    high-fat, 28
Dumbbells, 4, 240, 242, 244, 246
    controlled lifting of, 50
    weight of, 30, 120

Elbow joints, 148–49
"Enriched" flour, 87
Exercise. *See* Cardiovascular exercise;
    TONING EXERCISES

Fat, *vii,* 29, 58
    discussed, 21–22
    plan for week, 24
    See also Fat Budget; Fat-free foods; Fat
        grams; Low-fat diet
Fat Budget, 7–8, 10–12, 21, 29, 39, 93
The Fat Counter (Pocket Books), 8, 39
Fat-free foods, 58, 67
Fat grams, 7–8, 21, 39, 76
Fiber, *vii–ix,* 76, 87, 141, 184
    discussed, 129–31
    minimum daily amount, 142
    plan for week, 132
Fiber Goal, 137
Fish, 94, 178
Focus plan, *vii–viii*
Folic acid, 172, 173
Food Group Servings, 7, 10–11
Food labels, 21, 41, 70
    and fiber, 130, 137
    "hydrogenated vegetable oil," 40
    and sugar, 183, 185
Fruit, 75, 76, 85, 129, 130, 183
    canned, 175
    vitamins in, 165–66

Glutes muscles, 59
    See also Buttocks; Hips
Grains, 129, 130, 165, 166
Grape Nuts, 75

Hamburgers, 93
Hamstrings (rear thigh muscles), 15, 77
    stretch, 200
    toning exercises, 220–21, 222–23, 224–25,
        226–27, 232–33
HDLs (high-density lipoproteins), 40, 46, 47
Heart disease, 39–40, 66, 176, 184
    and fiber, 129, 130
    and LDL/HDL ratio, 46
    TFAs and, 52
Hips, 77, 95
    stretches, 201, 202
    toning exercise, 228–29
Honey, 76, 193
Hydrogenated vegetable oil, 40–41
Hydrogenation, 40

Immune system, 29
Insoluble fibers, 130–31
Insulin, 76
Iron, 141, 165–66, 172, 173, 178

Labels. *See* Food labels
Laxatives, 136
LDLs (low-density lipoproteins), 40, 46
Leg muscles, 185
Legumes, 94, 130
Lentils, 129

About the Authors

KATHY SMITH is a longtime leader in the fitness industry. She has touched millions of people by providing information on health, fitness, and nutrition. Kathy is the creator of twenty fitness videos that have topped the *Billboard* bestseller charts for more than twelve years. Her multimedia weight-management system, "WalkFit," proved so popular it has become an industry unto itself. It led to Kathy's writing the book *Kathy Smith's WalkFit for a Better Body,* as well as to the creation of an audiocassette series. She is a veteran fitness correspondent of NBC's *Today* show, ABC's *Good Morning America,* and Whittle Communications' *Special Reports TV*. Her "Pregnancy Workout" video was praised by the American Film Institute, the National Education Association, and *Billboard* magazine. Her involvement in nonprofit organizations includes serving on the board of directors of the Women's Sports Foundation (WSF) and the Earth Communications Office. In conjunction with WSF, Kathy created the Katie and Perrie Fund to promote the development of sports and fitness programs for girls ages five to nine. She lives with her husband and two daughters in California.

SUZANNE SCHLOSBERG is the coauthor of *Fitness For Dummies* (IDG Books, 1996) and the author of *The Ultimate Workout Log* (Houghton Mifflin, 1993). She is a contributing editor to *Health* and *Women's Sports and Fitness* magazines, and she writes regularly for *Shape*. Her work also has appeared in *Cooking Light,* the *Los Angeles Times, Men's Fitness, Outside,* and *Walking*.

Send inquiries to: Kathy Smith Lifestyles
                    P.O. Box 491433
                    Los Angeles, CA 90049

ADULT READING SERIES

Challenger

Teacher's Manual

FOR BOOK 8

COREA MURPhY

ISBN 0-88336-795-5

© 1989
New Readers Press
Publishing Division of Laubach Literacy International
Box 131, Syracuse, New York 13210

Printed in the United States of America

Cover design by Chris Steenwerth

9 8 7 6 5 4 3 2

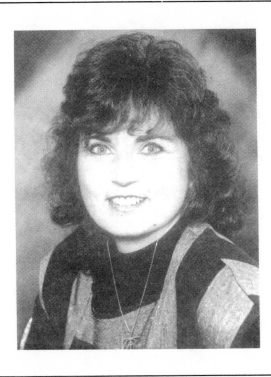

About the Author

Corea Murphy has worked in the field of education since the early 1960s. In addition to classroom and tutorial teaching, Ms. Murphy has developed language arts curriculum guides for public high schools, conducted curriculum and effectiveness workshops, and established an educational program for residents in a drug rehabilitation facility.

Ms. Murphy became interested in creating a reading series for older students when she began working with illiterate adults and adolescents in the early 1970s. The **Challenger Adult Reading Series** is the result of her work with these students.

In a very real sense, these students contributed greatly to the development of this reading series. Their enthusiasm for learning to read and their willingness to work hard provided inspiration, and their many helpful suggestions influenced the content of both the student books and the teacher's manuals.

It is to these students that the **Challenger Adult Reading Series** is dedicated with the hope that others who wish to become good readers will find this reading program both helpful and stimulating.

A special note of gratitude is also extended to Kay Koschnick, Christina Jagger, and Mary Hutchison of New Readers Press for their work and support in guiding this series to completion.

Table of Contents

Introduction to the *Challenger* Series

Challenger Adult Reading Series is an eight-book program of reading, writing, and reasoning skills designed to meet the needs of adult and adolescent students. It takes students from the beginning stages of reading to the critical reading, writing, and reasoning skills associated with the latter ninth grade level. The first four books in this series emphasize "learning to read." Beginning with the fifth book, the emphasis shifts to "reading to learn."

Each book in this controlled vocabulary series contains twenty lessons, plus reviews. Each lesson includes a reading selection and a variety of exercises and activities.

The reading selections in the odd-numbered books are generally fiction pieces. Books 1 and 3 contain light-hearted stories about adult characters who get caught up in a variety of situations. Most reading selections in Books 5 and 7 are minimally adapted well-known works of fiction.

The reading selections in the even-numbered books are engaging nonfiction pieces. The selections in Books 2 and 4 are generally similar to topics found in encyclopedias. Most selections in Books 6 and 8 are adaptations from highly-respected works of nonfiction. These selections enable students to broaden the scope of their knowledge.

Preceding each reading selection in the odd-numbered books is a word chart that introduces new words according to a specific phonics principle. In Books 1 and 3, these words appear frequently in both the reading selections and the exercises. In Books 5 and 7, the words from these charts are the basis for dictionary work and other word study exercises.

The wide variety of exercises and activities helps students develop their reading, writing, and reasoning skills and increase their basic knowledge. Comprehension exercises based on the reading selections focus on the development of literal, inferential, and critical reading skills. Also, the comprehension exercises in Books 5 through 8 introduce or reinforce various concepts associated with literary understanding.

Word study exercises are designed to increase the students' vocabulary and further develop their reading and reasoning skills. These exercises vary from simple word associations to classifying, sequencing, and categorizing exercises, analogies, vocabulary reviews, activities which emphasize using context clues, those which require using dictionaries and other reference materials, and several types of puzzles.

Students are eased into writing. Early in the series, exercises focus on writing at the sentence level and are designed to simultaneously improve spelling, sentence structure, and students' skill in expressing themselves clearly. Most lessons in Books 5 through 8 include at least one exercise in which the student must write responses in complete sentences or brief paragraphs. The individual lesson notes in this manual offer suggestions of topics to be considered for additional writing assignments. Although *Challenger* is primarily a reading series, teachers should encourage their students to understand that writing is an essential aspect of literacy.

The review lessons of Books 1 through 5 contain indexes of the words introduced in the preceding lessons. Word indexes are included in the Teacher's Manuals for Books 6 through 8. These indexes can be used in developing various reinforcement activities and vocabulary reviews.

The books also include periodic reviews. The last review in each book can be used as a diagnostic tool to determine the appropriate placement for students using this program. An accuracy rate of 85% or better on the final reviews indicates that a student is ready for the next book.

Significant Educational Features

Wide Learning Suitability/ Minimal Instructional Needs

This series has been tested successfully with students in many different types of instructional settings:

- Secondary remedial reading programs
- Secondary special education programs
- Adult volunteer literacy programs
- ABE, pre-GED, and GED programs
- Community college reading programs
- Educational programs in correctional institutions
- Tutorial programs for employees who wish to develop literacy skills in order to advance in their chosen occupations

Because both adults and older teens develop their skills more effectively when they assume a high degree of responsibility for their learning development, the lessons in the *Challenger* series have been designed so that they can be completed by students with only minimal instruction from the teacher.

An Integrated Approach

These books integrate reading, writing, and reasoning activities. The words introduced in each lesson provide the organizing principle for this integration. Through frequently seeing and using these words in reading, writing, and reasoning activities which are repeated in design but varied in content, students are better able to understand and apply what they have learned to a variety of situations. The thoroughness of this integrated approach enables students to begin each new lesson with greater mastery and confidence.

Sequenced Skill Building

Each lesson builds upon skills and content which students have worked with in previous lessons. Students experience a sense of progress because they quickly learn to apply their skills to new situations.

Students are continually challenged by the increased breadth and difficulty of each lesson, through which their reading progress is reflected. Generally, each reading selection is slightly longer than the previous one. In addition, the content, vocabulary, and sentence structure in the reading selections gradually become more sophisticated and demanding. The exercises, too, capitalize on students' increasing proficiency. Building on students' current skill level, the exercises gradually expand the students' knowledge in a spiral-like fashion—both broadening and deepening their abilities in the various skill areas.

Highly Motivating Material

For the past ten years, this series has been used with adult and adolescent populations for which it is designed. Students comment that many characteristics of this reading program help to hold their interest in their efforts to become more proficient readers. The characteristics they most frequently cite include:

- the exceptionally motivating reading selections
- the mature presentation and diversity of material
- the information presented in each lesson
- the emphasis on using reasoning powers
- the challenge of increasingly difficult materials
- the success and confidence the *Challenger* books generate

Comprehensive Teacher's Manuals

The comprehensive teacher's manuals offer practical suggestions about procedures and techniques for working with students. Individual lesson notes in the manuals present objectives, guidelines, and suggestions for specific activities in each lesson. A complete answer key for each lesson also appears in each manual.

> Although it is recognized that there are students of both sexes, for the sake of clarity and simplicity, we chose to use the pronouns *he, him,* and *his* throughout this book.

SCOPE AND SEQUENCE: BOOK 8

Vocabulary / Lesson	1	2	3	4	5	R	6	7	8	9	10	R	11	12	13	14	15	R	16	17	18	19	20	R
1. Learn unfamiliar vocabulary	★	★	★	★	★	★	★	★	★	★	★	★	★	★	★	★	★	★	★	★	★	★	★	★
2. Infer word meanings from context clues	☆	☆	☆	☆	☆	★	★	★	☆	☆	☆	★	☆	☆	★	★	★	★	★	★	★	☆	☆	★
3. Identify definitions/descriptions of terms	★	★	★	★	★	★	★	☆	★			★	★			☆	★	★	★	★		☆		★
4. Identify synonyms	★		★	★	★	★				★			★	★							☆	☆	☆	
5. Identify antonyms		☆	★			★						★				☆			★	★	☆			★
6. Complete word associations			★	★					★						★	☆						☆		
7. Complete analogies		☆	☆		☆	☆		☆	★	☆	☆	★					★							
8. Increase understanding of prefixes & suffixes	☆			☆		☆		☆			☆		☆	☆			☆			☆	☆			☆
9. Review homonyms																								
10. Learn etymological origins		☆							☆			☆	☆	☆			☆							☆
11. Complete word puzzles														☆					☆					
12. Use word families correctly															☆			☆						
13. Form/use compound words				☆		☆			☆			☆							☆					
14. Learn/review idioms, sayings, & proverbs																							☆	

Literary Understanding / Lesson	1	2	3	4	5	R	6	7	8	9	10	R	11	12	13	14	15	R	16	17	18	19	20	R
1. Identify/interpret characters' actions, motivations, feelings, and qualities	★				★	★		★	☆		★		☆		★	★	★		★	★	★	★		
2. Infer/interpret author's purpose/attitude	★								☆				☆					☆		★		★		
3. Predict/describe future/alternative events	★			★	★	★			★	★	☆					★	★	★	★	★		★	★	
4. Interpret poetry						★				★								★				★	★	
5. Compare/contrast points of view						★			☆		☆		☆		☆	☆	☆	★	☆	☆		★	★	
6. Interpret figurative language					★	★			★	★	★					★	★			★		★		
7. Relate to characters' motivations & feelings	☆				★	★			★	★	★					☆	☆		★		☆	★		
8. Identify setting					☆	☆	☆		☆	☆	☆		☆			☆	☆			☆			☆	☆
9. Interpret drama																				★				
10. Identify literary genres	☆																			☆		☆	☆	

Key: ★ = Primary emphasis ☆ = Secondary emphasis ☆ = Integrated with other skills

Comprehension

Lesson	1	2	3	4	5	R	6	7	8	9	10	R	11	12	13	14	15	R	16	17	18	19	20	R
1. Read selections independently	★	★	★	★	★	★	★	★	★	★	★	★	★	★	★	★	★	★	★	★	★	★	★	★
2. Complete exercises independently	★	★	★	★	★	★	★	★	★	★	★	★	★	★	★	★	★	★	★	★	★	★	★	★
3. Identify words using context clues	★	★	★	★	★	★	★	★	★	★	★	★	★	★	★	★	★	★	★	★	★	★	★	★
4. Improve listening comprehension	☆	☆	☆	☆	☆	☆	☆	☆	☆	☆	☆	☆	☆	☆	☆	☆	☆	☆	☆	☆	☆	☆	☆	☆
5. Improve oral reading skills	☆	☆	☆	☆	☆	☆	☆	☆	☆	☆	☆	☆	☆	☆	☆	☆	☆	☆	☆	☆	☆	☆	☆	☆
6. Develop literal comprehension skills:																								
—Recall details	☆	☆	☆	☆	☆		☆	☆	☆	☆	☆		☆	☆	☆	☆	☆		☆	☆	☆	☆	☆	
—Locate specific information	☆	☆	☆	☆	☆		☆	☆	☆	☆	☆		☆	☆	☆	☆	☆		☆	☆	☆	☆	☆	
—Establish sequence of events	★						☆	☆									★							
7. Develop inferential comprehension skills:																								
—Support statements with appropriate details	★	★	★	★	★	★	★	★	★	★	★	★	★	★	★	★	★	★	★	★	★	★	★	★
—Infer word meanings from context clues	★	★	★	★	★	★	★	★	★	★	★	★	★	★	★	★	★	★	★	★	★	★	★	★
—Infer information from readings & exercises	★	★	★	★	★	★	★	★	★	★	★	★	★	★	★	★	★	★	★	★	★	★	★	★
—Draw conclusions based on reading	★	★	★	★	★	★	★	★	★	★	★	★	★	★	★	★	★	★	★	★	★	★	★	★
—Compare/contrast points of view		★	★				☆	☆	★				★	☆	★					★	★		☆	
—Relate examples to ideas	☆				★	★	★	★		☆	☆		☆		☆			★		☆		★		
—Use context clues to fill in missing words	☆				☆			☆	★	☆				★		☆		★	☆	★		★		
—Identify/interpret humor																								
—Identify/infer cause & effect relationships					☆	☆	★	☆		☆		★	★			☆	☆			☆	★			
—Organize information in outline form							☆							☆					★					
—Classify words under topic headings	★					☆															★			
—Distinguish between fact & opinion														★			☆					☆		
8. Develop applied comprehension skills:																								
—Draw conclusions based on personal experience	★	★	★	★	★	★	★	★	★	★	★	★	★	★	★	★	★	★	★	★	★	★	★	★
—Relate reading to personal experience	★	★								★	★	★						★		★		★	★	
—Design a bar graph		★										★												
—Draw a diagram										★		★		★										
9. Learn/review basic factual information	☆	☆	☆	☆	☆	☆	☆	☆	☆	☆	☆	☆	☆	☆	☆	☆	☆	☆	☆	☆	☆	☆	☆	☆
10. Locate/infer information from:																								
—maps		★										★												
—editorial cartoons			★																					
—charts & graphs							★				★	★											★	
—diagrams						☆															☆		★	★

Key: ★ = Primary emphasis   ☆ = Secondary emphasis   ☆ = Integrated with other skills

Writing	1	2	3	4	5	R	6	7	8	9	10	R	11	12	13	14	15	R	16	17	18	19	20	R
1. Write sentence or paragraph answers to questions	★	★	★	★	★	★	★	★	★	★	★		★	★	★	★	★	★	★	★	★	★	★	☆
2. Form a reasoned opinion	★	★	★	★	★	★	★	★	★	★	★		★	★	★	★	★	★	★	★	★	★	★	☆
3. Support statements with details	★	★	★	★	★	★	★	★	★	★	★		★	★	★	★	★	★	★	★	★	★	★	
4. Copy words accurately	☆	☆	☆	☆	☆	☆	☆	☆	★	☆	☆	☆	☆	☆	☆	☆	☆	☆	☆	☆	☆	☆	☆	☆
5. Spelling:																								
—Spell words with greater accuracy	☆		☆	☆	☆	☆	☆	☆	☆	☆	☆	☆	☆	☆	☆	☆	☆	☆	☆	☆	☆	☆	☆	☆
—Spell homonyms correctly																	★							
—Identify misspelled words				☆				☆																
—Review singular & plural words		★																			★			
6. Write contrasting statements	☆		☆	☆																☆				
7. Write dialogue																								

Note: Specific suggestions for additional writing assignments appear in the individual lesson notes and in Chapter 5 of this manual.

Study Skills	1	2	3	4	5	R	6	7	8	9	10	R	11	12	13	14	15	R	16	17	18	19	20	R
1. Increase concentration	☆	☆	☆	☆	☆	☆	☆	☆	☆	☆	☆	☆	☆	☆	☆	☆	☆	☆	☆	☆	☆	☆	☆	☆
2. Skim selection to locate information	☆	☆	☆	☆	☆	☆	☆	☆	☆	☆	☆	☆	☆	☆	☆	☆	☆	☆	☆	☆	☆	☆	☆	☆
3. Apply reasoning skills to exercises:																								
—context clues	☆	☆	☆	☆	☆	☆	★	★	☆	☆	☆	☆	☆	☆	☆	☆	☆	★	☆	☆	☆	☆	☆	☆
—process of elimination	☆	☆	☆	☆	☆	☆	☆	☆	☆	☆	☆	☆	☆	☆	☆	☆	☆	☆	☆	☆	☆	☆	☆	☆
—"intelligent guessing"	☆	☆	☆	☆	☆	☆	☆	☆	☆	☆	☆	☆	☆	☆	☆	☆	☆	☆	☆	☆	☆	☆	☆	☆
4. Use a dictionary:																								
—to look up word meanings	☆	☆	☆	☆	☆	☆	☆	☆	☆	☆	☆	☆	☆	☆	☆	☆	☆	☆	☆	☆	☆		☆	☆
—to learn word origins	☆											☆												
—to learn plural forms of words								☆								☆								
—to form compound words																								
5. Use reference materials to find factual/ geographical information	☆				★		☆						☆	☆	☆				☆	☆			☆	☆

Key: ★ = Primary emphasis ☆ = Secondary emphasis ☆ = Integrated with other skills

1. Introduction to Book 8

The format of Book 8 corresponds to the one used in earlier even-numbered books in the *Challenger* series. Book 8 introduces relatively few new words and concepts in order to give students the opportunity to thoroughly review and reinforce vocabulary and reasoning skills and further develop their reading comprehension.

The readings for Book 8 are, for the most part, nonfiction selections which have been minimally adapted from works of widely-acclaimed writers. Experience indicates that motivation and self-esteem are bolstered when students are made aware of this fact. Adult students should also be made aware that the GED Test includes brief, nonfiction passages with accompanying questions. In working with the readings in Book 8, adults often become increasingly confident of their ability to achieve this long-range educational goal.

A review appears after every five lessons. These reviews provide students with additional opportunities to review words and concepts. They also help students develop the habit of referring to previous lessons for the correct answers to some of the questions.

Book 8 is generally used by students who have completed Book 7 in this series. Book 8 is also appropriate for use with students who score in the range of 8.5 and above on standardized reading achievement tests. The final review in Book 7 can also be used as a diagnostic tool. An accuracy rate of 85% or better for this review indicates that students are ready for Book 8.

Students who use this book should be given as many opportunities for oral reading practice as time permits. This practice helps to develop confidence, enjoyment, and interest in reading.

Book 8 builds upon procedures and practices emphasized in the earlier books in this series. Thus, you may find it worthwhile to look through the manual notes for some of these books.

Scheduling Considerations

Book 8 works well in a classroom setting. The most progress is achieved when students work with *Challenger* a minimum of 45 minutes two or three times a week. Students can work independently, in a group, or with a partner. When working with other students, they receive the support and stimulation from one another that makes learning more enjoyable. Also, the more advanced students can assume much of the responsibility for giving explanations and leading reinforcement activities, which in turn reinforces their own reading skills. Experience indicates that less advanced students usually benefit from peer instruction provided that you are available to supply any necessary clarifications.

The Lesson Components

Later chapters of this manual outline the principles and procedures that form the foundation of this reading series. The major components of the lessons in Book 8 are briefly described below.

Words for Study

This section, which precedes the reading selection in each lesson, lists words in the lesson that appear for the first time in this series. As was the case in the earlier books, these words appear in the same order and form in which they initially appear in the lesson. This gives students additional practice in pronouncing word endings accurately.

The Reading Selection

The readings for Book 8 have been organized into four units: Appearances, Time, the Good Earth, and Change. Although a work of fiction has been included in each of these units, the emphasis is on nonfiction. Because some students still have difficulty distinguishing fiction from nonfiction, these terms should be mentioned when appropriate. You will also have the occasion to review the terms *biography* and *autobiography*. Keep these reviews short and simple. Terminology is best understood when it is presented in small, repeated doses.

All initial readings, with the exception of the first lesson, are to be done as homework activities.

Understanding the Reading

The comprehension questions call for a variety of different responses: multiple choice, fill-in-the-blank, and complete sentence and paragraph responses. This variety gives students practice with formats that appear on both job-placement tests and the GED Test—two exams that many students using this book may well encounter.

Most of the adaptations or excerpts in Book 8 encourage critical thinking. By no means should the comprehension questions be considered the final word on the topics and themes discussed in the readings. As often as possible, regard the comprehension exercises as a point of departure for further exploration.

Other Exercises

A wide variety of exercises has been included to help students improve their recall, increase their vocabulary, and develop their reasoning abilities. As often as seems appropriate, draw the students' attention to the fact that reasoning is an essential part of reading. Help them develop such patterns as using the process of elimination, making intelligent guesses, using the dictionary, and referring to previous lessons when completing these exercises.

A score of 80% or higher should be considered satisfactory on these exercises. If students consistently score below this figure, take some time to help them pinpoint the problem. Generally, they are trying to complete the exercises too rapidly.

Because students are encouraged to learn from their mistakes, they should not be penalized for making them. If you work in a school which gives report cards, it is strongly recommended that evaluations be based on corrected work and overall progress rather than on students' initial efforts. In no way does this practice encourage typical reading students to be careless in completing their homework. Rather they usually become more interested in reading than in report cards, they are more relaxed and patient with themselves in completing assignments, and they develop a more realistic definition of academic progress.

Reinforcement Activities

Suggestions and procedures for reinforcement activities for those words and concepts that give students difficulty are discussed in Chapter 4.

Writing Assignments

Student writing is discussed in Chapter 5. It is recommended that students working in Book 8 complete weekly writing assignments of 350-600 words in addition to the writing that is required to complete the exercises in the individual lessons. Suggestions for writing assignments are given in the individual lesson notes. It is also recommended that students working in Book 8 keep a journal in which they briefly record their responses to the readings or class discussions.

The Lesson Format

The procedure for each lesson should be as consistent as possible.

1. Students go over the writing assignment if one was given and review the work in the previous lesson first. This includes discussing the reading selection and correcting the exercises.

2. If time permits, students complete relevant reinforcement activities. The nature and scope of these activities are determined by the needs of your students and how often you meet with them.

3. Students preview the next lesson, which is usually assigned for homework.

Individual Lesson Notes

Lesson notes for each individual lesson appear in Chapter 7 of this manual. These notes contain suggestions and procedures for specific items in each lesson.

Answer Key

An answer key for all the exercises in each lesson of Book 8 follows the lesson notes.

Word Indexes

The word indexes at the back of this manual contain lists of words that are introduced to this series in each unit of Book 8. There is also a master list of all the words introduced in this book. These lists are helpful when developing reinforcement activities. Students may also want to consult these lists periodically.

The next three chapters give suggestions for preparing and teaching the lessons and selecting reinforcement activities.

2. Preparing to Teach

The following suggestions are based on the author's experiences and those of other teachers who have used these books. You may find that your own situation renders some of these suggestions either impractical or impossible to implement in your classroom. It is hoped, however, that most of these suggestions can be modified to meet your particular needs.

How Often to Use Challenger

In general, it is recommended that teachers use Challenger with students two or three times a week for at least 45 minutes per session. If you meet five times a week with pre-GED students who are eager to pass the tests and have time outside the classroom to complete homework assignments, you may want to use Challenger every day.

If you meet five times a week with an adult or adolescent reading class that does not have a specific task such as GED preparation to motivate them, the recommended schedule is to focus on the lessons three times a week and devote the other two class sessions to activities which reinforce or enrich material presented in the lessons. Suggestions about these reinforcement activities appear in Chapter 4.

It is important that students recognize the need to work with Challenger regularly. This is often an issue for students in volunteer programs or institutions in which class attendance is not mandatory. Whatever the situation, if a student chooses to attend class on a highly infrequent basis, tell him politely but frankly that there is little point in his attending at all because he's not giving himself a chance to make any significant progress.

If only one class meeting a week is possible, try to schedule this class for 90 minutes to two hours. Also, have the students complete two lessons and, if appropriate, a writing activity for homework. When the students look at you as if you were crazy, show them that by completing a few components of the lessons each day, they will not only be able to do the work, but also reinforce what they are learning. Sports and music are helpful analogies because most students know that both require daily practice.

The Lesson Format

After the first class, which of course involves no homework review, the procedure for each lesson is basically the same. The overview below gives you an idea of what happens during each class. More detailed procedures for this work appear in later chapters of this manual.

1. **Writing assignment.** If students have been given a writing assignment, begin the class by letting them share their work in pairs or small groups. Chapter 5 gives details on writing assignments.

2. **Homework review.** Discuss the reading selection to make sure students have understood it and to give them a chance to react to the reading. Then go over the comprehension questions and the other exercises and have students make any necessary corrections.

3. **Reinforcement activity.** If no writing assignment was given and if time permits, have the students do one or more reinforcement activities. See Chapter 4 for suggestions about reinforcement activities.

4. **Homework preview.** Go over the Words for Study listed at the beginning of the lesson. Introduce the reading selection and call attention to any special features that may be new or confusing. Have students quickly preview the individual exercises for anything they don't understand.

Following this general procedure on a fairly consistent basis helps students because they tend to feel more relaxed and work better when they have a sense of routine. Modifications in the procedure should be made only when they will enhance students' reading development.

Just as you encourage students to see homework assignments as daily workouts, encourage them to see class time as a daily workout, also. These lessons should not be seen as achievement tests but rather as opportunities to move students smoothly toward their reading goals. Students do not have to demonstrate mastery of the material in one lesson in order to go on to the next lesson. Mastery will come with consistent practice.

It is crucial for teachers to think in terms of improvement rather than mastery because students using these books often want to add a fourth component to the lesson format—rationalizing and/or lamenting their mistakes. This uses up valuable classroom time and, if allowed a foothold, will result in students' giving up and dropping out. Students must learn to perceive their mistakes as a natural and helpful part of the learning process. They can learn this only by your gentle but firm reminder that consistent practice is the key to mastery.

Remember that both adult and adolescent reading students tend to be overly sensitive to mistakes in their work. In most cases, they firmly believe that if they hadn't made so many mistakes in the first place, they wouldn't have to be working in these books. For example, a woman in her mid-twenties who decided to quit class explained her reason this way: "My teacher told me that it was all right to make mistakes, but every time I had one in my work she would kind of close her eyes and shake her head like I should have learned all this in the fourth grade." Teachers must think and act in terms of improvement rather than mastery and regard mistakes as natural and helpful.

Do not expect to know at the outset how much time to allot to each segment of the lesson. Understanding exactly how to pace the lessons takes time. By paying attention to students' responses and rate of accuracy, you will gradually learn how to schedule the lessons so that students improve their reading and writing skills in a relaxed but efficient manner.

Preparing the Lessons

In preparing the lessons, develop the habit of following this procedure:

1. Familiarize yourself with the lesson students are to work on that day.
2. Review the appropriate lesson notes in Chapter 7 of this manual for suggestions to help you teach the lesson. Go over the appropriate answers in the Answer Key as well.
3. Review any notes you took after the preceding class in which you jotted down vocabulary words or writing difficulties that students need to review. Teacher notetaking is discussed in Chapter 6 of this manual.
4. Decide upon any reinforcement activities you may want to use and complete any preparation needed. Suggestions for reinforcement activities are given in Chapter 4.
5. Skim the lesson to be assigned for homework and the appropriate lesson notes so you can introduce the reading selection and answer any questions students may have about the exercises.

Last and most important, you need to prepare yourself mentally and emotionally for the class. If possible, take several minutes before the students' arrival to unwind from the previous activities of the day. As a general rule, how well the lesson goes is determined by how relaxed and focused you are on the work. As the teacher, your main function is to serve as a smooth bridge between the student and the lesson material. Your own patience and concentration will determine how helpful this "bridge" is.

The Teacher-Student Relationship

Making sure that you are relaxed for the lesson also contributes to the development of a good working relationship with your students. Adolescent or adult reading students rely heavily on your support and encouragement.

It is helpful to remember that most of us, as we grow older, learn to fake or avoid situations in which we feel inadequate. We prefer habits and routines that are familiar and give us some sense of security. Adolescent or adult reading students have entered into a situation in which they can neither avoid (unless they give up) nor fake their way through the material. They are to be admired for having put themselves in this situation. Unless they are extremely motivated or thick-skinned, they must feel a sense of support from you or they will eventually drop out, because exposing their lack of knowledge just gets too painful after a while.

In addition, completing the lessons in these books *is* hard work. No matter how much progress is being made, virtually all students experience a sense of frustration at one time or another. Your encouragement will help them to get through these gloomy periods when they are ready to throw in the towel.

Suggestions for a Good Working Rapport

The following are suggestions to help you consider how best to develop a good working relationship with your students.

- Strive for naturalness in your voice and mannerisms. Some teachers unconsciously treat reading students as if they were mental invalids or victims of a ruthless society. A condescending or pitying approach does not help students become better readers.
- Greet the students pleasantly and spend a few minutes in casual conversation before you actually begin work. As a rule, do not allow this conversation to exceed five minutes. Students will take their cue from you. If you encourage conversing rather than working, they will be more than willing to oblige.
- Participate fully in this pre-lesson conversation and listen attentively to the students' remarks. Often you can later refer to these remarks when you are helping students to understand a vocabulary word or a point in the reading selection. Not only do they appreciate the fact that you actually were listening to them, but also they begin to make connections with the material they are studying.
- Use a phrase such as "Shall we get started?" to indicate that it is time to begin the lesson. A consistent use of such transitional statements helps the students feel more comfortable with both you and the class routine.
- If possible, work at an uncluttered table rather than at desks. Try to have straight-backed, cushioned chairs since physical comfort makes developing a good relationship easier.
- Be sure to use positive reinforcement during the lesson. Remind students of the progress they are making. When a student is particularly discouraged, do this in a concrete way. For example, show him how many pages of work he has completed, or have him look at his composition book to see all the writing he has done.
- Develop the habit of wishing students a good day or a good evening as they leave the class. This is especially important if both you and the students have had a rough session. The students, particularly adolescents, need to know that you don't carry personal grudges.

Classroom Supplies

For each class, students need to bring their *Challenger* book, their composition book, and a pen or pencil. The use of the composition book—a slim, loose-leaf binder with wide-lined paper—is discussed in Chapter 5.

You need your own copy of *Challenger*, any notes and reinforcement activities pertaining to the lesson, a few sheets of blank paper for notes, and a pen. A pen is recommended because students can spot your marginal notes and corrections more easily. Avoid red ink as it is frequently associated with too many bad memories.

Have a dictionary and, if possible, a set of encyclopedias, a globe or an atlas within easy reach. The encyclopedia and the dictionary are valuable resources because they provide pictures and additional information about many of the words, people, and events mentioned in the reading selections and exercises. Be prepared to teach students how to use these resources. Do not assume that students working at a Book 8 reading level are familiar with them.

A globe or world map is helpful because it can make the facts presented in the lessons more meaningful to students. For example, in Lesson 2, Exercise 5, the students complete an exercise about the South Pacific. A small map is included in the workbook. It is very helpful to find this area on a globe or world map to give students a better idea of the location and size of the area.

Encourage students to research additional information as often as their interest, abilities, and time permit and give them all the assistance you can when they need help. These mini-research experiences help students feel more competent when searching for information.

A Summary of Do's

1. Do try to schedule at least two classes each week which meet at a regularly-appointed time.
2. Do take time to develop a consistent lesson format that will work well for your students.
3. Do perceive your students' work in terms of improvement rather than mastery.
4. Do take time to prepare for each class.
5. Do give yourself a few moments to relax before each class.
6. Do develop a good working relationship with students because it is essential to their reading progress.
7. Do make sure that the environment in which you teach is as conducive to good learning as possible.
8. Do have reference and resource materials available, if possible.
9. Do give the students positive reinforcement during the lessons.

3. Teaching the Lessons

In this chapter, suggestions are given for teaching the main components of each lesson. These components include the word study, the reading selection, the exercises, correcting the homework, and the homework preview.

Word Study

The *Challenger* series places a great deal of emphasis on learning and/or reviewing word meanings since a major obstacle to reading development is a poor vocabulary. It has been estimated that only about 2,000 words account for 99% of everything we say. To be a proficient reader, however, one must be familiar with far more than 2,000 words. Thus, most of the exercises which follow each reading selection focus on vocabulary development.

Keep in mind that the *Challenger* series is a controlled vocabulary series. When students wish to know how the words listed in the Words for Study at the beginning of each lesson have been selected, inform them that these words are appearing for the first time in the series. Most of the other words in each lesson have appeared earlier in the series.

Students not only find the concept of a controlled vocabulary interesting, but some interpret this concept in interesting ways. For example, one student who was experiencing difficulty with a synonym exercise in Book 8 remarked: "Well, you can't expect me to know words that were studied in Book 7!"

Behind this statement is a conviction shared by many reading students that once you've studied a word, you should never have to study it again. Unfortunately, this is not true. Words are learned through repetition, practice, and using the dictionary. Do not assume that your students know this. Simply remind them, when appropriate, that a good reading vocabulary is necessary for good reading and that they will encounter a word in various types of exercises so that they can truly master its meaning.

The best way to encourage your students as they complete the many vocabulary development exercises is to demonstrate an interest in language yourself. This does not mean that you have to use a lot of "fancy" words when talking to your students. What it does mean is that you do not approach vocabulary study as if it were something to be merely endured.

Here are a few suggestions for making vocabulary study more interesting for students:

1. Have students pronounce the Words for Study in the next lesson during the homework preview. Most words will not give them any trouble. By pronouncing the unfamiliar ones, students will gain confidence in their ability to learn the word, and confidence often leads to interest.

2. Encourage students to develop the habit of paying attention to word endings. Words listed in the Words for Study appear in the same form in which they appear in the reading. For example, notice that in Lesson 2, *civilized* is listed. Emphasis on accurate pronunciations of endings will help students with both their reading and writing.

3. When time permits, spend a few minutes in casual conversation about some of the words. Using Lesson 3 as an example, you may wish to talk about two ways in which the word *media* can be used, or have students identify the root in *elimination*, or help them trace the origin of *fantasy* in a good dictionary. Occasional discussion of words helps students to see them as more than just a string of letters.

4. Take time during discussions of the readings to highlight vocabulary and/or language features. In Lesson 1, for instance, students enjoy reading the Virginia newspaper account of April 1900 aloud and then substituting more modern phrasing for some of the words in the article. These brief discussions help students to see that language patterns vary and that language is always changing.

5. Finally, strive to speak with expression. You needn't be a Broadway star, but a little ham goes a long way.

The Reading Selections

The amount of time you allot to oral reading and discussion of the reading selections ultimately depends on both the needs of your students and how much class time you have with them.

Oral Reading

Having students read aloud at least part of the reading selection periodically gives you an opportunity to note their strengths and weaknesses and also to help them develop good oral reading habits. Some students are under the impression that good oral reading means that one reads as fast as one can. Remind these students that in oral reading one must always be conscious of the needs of the listeners.

Discussing the Reading

Have a general discussion of the reading selection to refresh students' memories and to make sure they have understood the reading. Then discuss their responses to the comprehension exercises.

To create an atmosphere in which the reading selections and student thoughts about them can be discussed with a sense of harmony and unity, consider these suggestions.

1. Plan questions that you want to ask in class. Be prepared, however, to put your planned questions aside when a spontaneous question arises in class.

2. Make sure students understand the basic ground rule of all good discussions: one person speaks at a time.

3. Encourage participation, but don't force it. Likewise, discourage students from monopolizing the discussion.

4. Keep the discussion focused.

5. Avoid asking "yes" and "no" questions. Discussions, like travel, should be broadening. "Yes" and "no" questions shut off discussion by being answerable in a single word. They also imply that the student should have reached a conclusion before the discussion has even started.

6. If students seem confused by your questions, rephrase them rather than repeating them word-for-word. This practice is not only courteous, but it also reminds students that there is usually more than one way to phrase an idea.

These suggestions represent the easier part of moderating a discussion. The harder part is staying out of the way. Your task as the moderator is to get students to react to each other's opinions and comments, not to dominate the discussion yourself.

It is essential to view discussions in the same way that you view the students' other work—in terms of improvement, or growth, instead of mastery. It takes time to develop a good discussion group in which participants can learn to really listen to each other and gain confidence to express themselves as genuinely as possible. Do not expect it to be otherwise.

Through these discussions, students begin to sense a relationship between the lesson material and their own lives. The relationships they have with you and the other students can become more relaxed and real. This, in turn, means that everyone learns better and faster.

The Exercises

In the exercises, students develop their reasoning abilities because they are required to think and infer, to use context clues, to practice the process of elimination, and to apply what they already know to new situations.

Three points that you should emphasize to students are accuracy, legibility, and completeness. They are to spell their responses correctly and legibly, and they are not to leave any item blank. Tell them to answer all questions to the best of their ability. Not only does learning thrive on corrected mistakes, but also much is to be said for the art of intelligent guessing.

Remind students to check over their homework after they have finished all the exercises to make sure they have answered all questions completely and accurately.

Allow enough time at the end of the class period for previewing the exercises that are to be completed for homework. It is important that students understand exactly what is expected of them, so don't rush this segment of the lesson.

You should spend a few minutes during the first class meeting with your students to review the importance of homework. Remember, some of your students haven't been in a school situation for quite a while, and they may need to be reminded of the importance of completing the assignments as well as they can.

Sometimes students try to complete the homework right after a full day's (or full night's) work, or just before going to bed, or while they are trying to fulfill other responsibilities. Suggest that they schedule a definite, 30-minute study time in quiet surroundings when they are not exhausted.

Make sure to present your ideas on how to develop better study habits in the form of suggestions. You are not stating policy; you are simply encouraging students to think about how they can better achieve their reading goals within the circumstances of their lives.

Correcting the Homework

Be sure you allow enough time to go over the homework with the students. You will probably need to observe your students and try out a few different schedules before you hit on the pace that works best for them. But once you establish the appropriate pace, consistency promotes good concentration and effective learning.

Of all the lesson segments—the words for study, the reading selection, and the exercises—the exercises should be covered most thoroughly. All the homework should be corrected. Remember that many patterns are being established. If students develop the habit of doing something incorrectly, they will have a hard time unlearning the procedure. Be sure to explain this to the students. Eventually, they adapt to this procedure because they see that the more they correct in the early stages, the less they have to correct later.

Too often, going over the homework can be nothing more than a dry, mechanical routine in which students simply read their answers. Not only does this deprive them of practice with the words and concepts they've been studying, but also it is unfair. Consciously or unconsciously, the students' efforts are being slighted if the homework critique is being done in a dreary, "what's-the-answer-to-number-2?" style.

Take your time and enjoy this part of the lesson. If opportunities arise for brief tangents in which items are related to life experiences or other bits of information, take advantage of them.

Above all, don't forget to express your appreciation for students' efforts. Your supportive remarks should be brief and spoken in a natural voice. Excessive praise is ultimately as counterproductive as no praise at all. Words of encouragement should stress the notion of progress because students are progressing as they complete each lesson.

The Homework Preview

During the homework preview the students note what to do in the next lesson, which they are to complete for homework. Begin by going over the words listed in the Words for Study. Then introduce the reading selection to give students an idea of what they will be reading about. It may be necessary to help students get into the habit of noting the title of the reading selection. They should understand that the title gives them a general idea of what the selection is about and helps to focus their attention.

Remind students to refer to the reading selection when they cannot recall an answer to a comprehension question. In many instances, they may need to make intelligent guesses based on information which is implied rather than stated directly.

At this point in their reading development, all students are able to skim through the exercises and ask questions about words and/or directions with no assistance from you. The individual lesson notes indicate those instances in which you may want to emphasize certain words or directions.

A Summary of Do's

1. Do take time when necessary to explain to students how vocabulary study, the reading selections, and exercises contribute to their reading development.

2. Do make vocabulary study as interesting as possible.

3. Do encourage students to have an attitude of growth rather than fixed opinions in their discussions.

4. Do remind students, when necessary, of the significant role that homework plays in reading development.

5. Do emphasize the need for thoroughness, correct spelling, and accuracy in completing each exercise.

6. Do strive for completeness and enthusiasm in the homework reviews.

7. Do support the students' progress by taking the time to point out growth they have demonstrated in their work.

8. Do allow enough time at the end of each lesson to go over the Words for Study, introduce the next reading selection, and preview the homework exercises.

4. Reinforcement Activities

As the term suggests, these activities are designed to reinforce the students' understanding and retention of the lesson material. All students and most teachers occasionally need a break in the routine. Reinforcement activities may throw your schedule off a bit, but it's worth it. Just make sure that you leave enough time at the end of the class period to preview the homework.

At this point in students' development, two types of activities are particularly helpful:

- Activities which reinforce vocabulary skills.

- Occasional, short exercises which focus on mechanical or usage errors most of your students repeatedly make in their compositions.

The types of activities you use and the frequency with which you use them depend on the needs of your students and how often you have an opportunity to meet with them. The suggestions in this section are based on activities that students have found both helpful and enjoyable. This list is by no means complete. Take some time to develop your own "bag of tricks." Through talking with other teachers, skimming puzzle magazines, and using your own imagination, you will soon have reinforcement activities for a variety of skills. Students, too, often recall helpful activities from their earlier schooling. In fact, some of the suggestions which follow come from students.

Word and Information Games

Students working at this level often enjoy games that are modeled after television shows such as *Jeopardy*. These activities take some time to prepare, but they are an excellent way to reinforce vocabulary and information presented in the lessons. Certainly you can prepare the questions, but having the students do it gives them an excellent opportunity to review the material.

Students can create their own *Jeopardy* games by preparing sets of questions based on the reading selections. They can also create sets of vocabulary questions. For example, all the answers in a category might begin with the prefix *pre-* or the letter *s*. Other appropriate categories include: State Capitals, Bodies of Water, U.S. Presidents, Roman Gods and Goddesses, Famous Inventors, Abbreviations, and so on.

Other game show formats can also be used. For example, students enjoy playing their own version of *Wheel of Fortune*. They also enjoy their version of *College Bowl* in which two teams compete against each other. In this game, the teacher can prepare the questions and act as the moderator.

Puzzles

Many puzzles and other activities can be found in puzzle magazines sold in most drugstores and supermarkets. You can create your own puzzles using these formats and vocabulary from past and current word indexes. The word indexes for Book 8 are at the back of this manual. If you have access to a computer, there is software available for creating crossword puzzles into which you can insert vocabulary words to be reinforced.

Spelling Bees or Drills

This activity is most helpful when a specific principle is emphasized; for example, selecting words which all contain a specific suffix or consonant blend, or which belong to the same word family. Again, the word indexes at the back of this manual can be helpful in developing these activities. Drills should be spontaneous, brief—10 words is usually sufficient—and informally presented. In other words, they should not resemble a quiz in which students demonstrate mastery. Rather they are an opportunity to help students to better understand certain language principles that are giving them difficulty.

Worksheets

One type of worksheet can focus on some principle that is giving students trouble, such as recognizing analogies, using context clues, or making inferences. A popular type of worksheet for context clue or vocabulary reinforcement is to collect sentences from a newspaper or magazine in which troublesome words you have been working with appear. Set them up in a fill-in-the-blank format for the students to complete as a group. As one student once remarked, "You mean people actually *do* use these words?" You might also tell students to be on the lookout for these words and have them bring to class examples that they find in their own reading.

Another type of worksheet can give students practice with some aspect of writing, such as capitalization or punctuation. For example, many students neglect to use commas after introductory clauses. You might prepare 10 sentences which begin with introductory clauses and have the students insert commas appropriately. Students find this type of introduction to grammar both tolerable and beneficial because it helps them to recall a rule they need for their own writing.

Enrichment Projects

Students can spend some time in the library seeking additional information about people or topics presented in the lessons and informally report their findings to the class. These reports can be given during the time set aside for reinforcement activities.

Any additional information that you can present also heightens the students' interest in the material. For example, for Lesson 1, you might invite an amateur magician to perform a few sleight-of-hand tricks for your students and then discuss how the illusions are accomplished. Other enrichment ideas are suggested in the individual lesson notes.

Activities Based on Student Needs

Occasionally students may have specific personal needs, such as filling out an application form or creating a resume, that can be fit comfortably into the lesson format as reinforcement activities if they tell you about them far enough in advance. However, reinforcement activities are to reinforce, not replace, the lessons. If students are spending most of their valuable class time hearing additional information about the reading selections or getting your assistance with personal needs, they may learn some interesting facts or get forms filled out, but they are not progressing in their reading development.

If you suspect that students are using reinforcement activities to avoid working on the lessons, you probably need to help them clarify their learning goals. Gently but firmly remind them that, in the long run, their reading and writing will progress more rapidly if they concentrate more on the lesson work and recognize that the primary reason for reinforcement activities is to do just that—reinforce.

A Note to the Teacher

Because it takes time to prepare many of these reinforcement activities, be sure to file them away for use with future students.

Also, do not pressure yourself to come up with something new every time you plan a reinforcement activity. It takes a few years to develop a solid file of activities.

A Summary of Do's and Don'ts

1. Do make sure the scheduled lesson time is not sacrificed for reinforcement activities.

2. Do involve the students in planning and creating reinforcement activities whenever possible.

3. Do plan and implement activities that address both the students' learning needs and their personal needs.

4. Do remember to save materials you develop for future use.

5. Don't foster a "here's-some-more-hard-work" attitude toward reinforcement activities. The students have just finished discussing a reading selection, reviewing their homework, and learning new material. If the reinforcement activities are to benefit them, they need a little more informality from you for this segment of the lesson.

6. Don't foster a "this-is-just-for-fun" attitude either. Students might not find the activities enjoyable. And you want students who do find them enjoyable to recognize that pleasure and learning can go hand in hand.

5. Writing

Because the major purpose of this reading series is to help students develop their reading skills, less emphasis has been placed on writing skills. Even though writing is an important skill, it is a distinct skill that requires a great deal of practice and instruction time. Generally, the writing activities included in Book 8 focus on clarity and completeness of expression, coherence of thought, basic grammar, and spelling. However, there are plentiful opportunities for students to express their own opinions and ideas in writing.

Why Writing Is Included

The teacher can assume that a student who has completed some of the books which precede Book 8 can write complete sentences and coherent paragraphs. These students will not be surprised at the exercises which involve writing in the later *Challenger* books.

Students who are new to this series may wonder why writing activities have been included in a reading series. When this is the case, take time to point out the following:

- Writing is part of literacy. To be literate, a person must be able to write as well as read.

- Writing helps students to formulate and express their thoughts more precisely. This type of thinking helps them to complete the other exercises more rapidly.

- The writing that students do in these lessons will help them with other types of writing they may want to do, such as letters, reports, and short paragraphs on job applications or resumes.

- Only through actually writing can students see that they are able to write.

Opportunities for Writing

In Book 8, an increasing emphasis is placed on content, rather than on the mechanics of writing. The reading comprehension questions require students to draw conclusions from inferences, to cite reasons to support their opinions, to give explanations for their answers, and to cite examples and details to support their responses. Exercises that focus on developing critical thinking include comparing and contrasting points of view, analyzing humor, writing optimistic and pessimistic statements, and interpreting poetry and cartoons. There are also opportunities for imaginative writing, including writing the endings to excerpts from longer works and describing what life might be like in a different time or place.

The individual lesson notes include many suggestions for writing assignments which can supplement the lessons as reinforcement activities. As stated in Chapter 1, it is recommended that weekly writing assignments of 350-600 words be given. However, the decision on how often to give writing assignments as homework should depend on the teacher's assessment of the students' time, personal needs, and capabilities. The key word is flexibility.

How to Handle Writing Assignments

When students have been given a writing assignment, have them share their work at the beginning of the next class session. Working in pairs or small groups, students can read their assignments aloud to one another and react to each other's writing on the basis of content and organization. Students can then exchange papers and act as editors or proofreaders, checking for mechanical problems such as missing words, spelling, capitalization, and punctuation. Give students the opportunity to revise their assignments before collecting them at the following class session.

When responding to these writing assignments, try to make positive comments as well as noting areas for improvement. Your reactions should be based more on the content, style, and organization of the writing than on the mechanical aspects.

It is recommended that students keep all writing assignments and journal entries in a slim, loose-leaf binder with wide-lined notebook paper. Composition books enable both the students and the teacher to quickly review student progress. Have them date their work. As the weeks and months progress, most students enjoy looking back now and then at all the writing they have done and see how much they have accomplished.

Like reading and vocabulary work, writing must be seen in terms of improvement rather than mastery. Most students read far better than they write. It is not uncommon for a student working in Book 8, for example, to write at a Book 5 level: simple sentences, few modifiers, and underdeveloped thoughts. The most common reason for this is lack of practice. Allow students to develop from their own starting points, making them aware of their strengths as well as helping them to work on their weaknesses. And don't forget to be patient.

Here are a few suggestions to consider in helping students with their writing:

- As often as possible, have students read their written responses or compositions aloud. Students usually enjoy doing this, and it gives them a chance to hear whether or not their writing makes sense. Insist on honest but courteously presented reactions from the other students.

- Occasionally, allot some class time to studying how the professional writers write. Use a reading selection from *Challenger* or an interesting magazine article. Help students analyze the piece of writing on the basis of content organization and style. Make sure students understand that the writing they are analyzing is more than a second, third, or fourth draft. Few students recognize the contribution editing makes in the writing process, and understanding this makes them feel less discouraged about their writing difficulties.

- With their permission, use writing from previous or present students as models to explain a particularly difficult writing assignment. Seeing the work of their peers often helps students realize that the teacher is not asking them to do the impossible.

- With their permission, compile a worksheet using sentences from student work which illustrate common mistakes. For example, a worksheet comprised of student-created run-on sentences is an excellent reinforcement activity. Students can work together in class to correct the errors and better understand how to avoid this particular writing problem.

- Provide the opportunity for students to publicly display their final drafts so other students can read them.

Dealing with Typical Writing Problems

Run-on Sentences

This situation demands consummate tact on your part because, invariably, the student thinks he has written a terrific sentence and is dismayed to learn that he has to divide it into three or four shorter sentences. Help him to see that, by using commas and periods wherever necessary, he helps readers to follow his thoughts more easily. To illustrate how punctuation helps the reader, have him read the sentence aloud, telling him to pause only at commas and to take a breath only at a period. If you prefer, you can demonstrate by reading his sentence to him. When he recognizes the value of punctuation marks, have him revise the run-on sentence as necessary. Be sure to commend him for his effort in helping to make his writing easier for readers to comprehend.

Omitted Words

When reading their sentences aloud, students are often surprised to see that they have omitted words. Remind them that many writers have this problem because the mind can think faster than the hand can write. Suggest that after they have written something, they should read it to themselves, pointing to each word as they encounter it. This strategy will help them learn to monitor their writing.

Confusing Sentences

When a student writes a sentence which is confusing, tell him you don't understand what he's trying to express and ask him to explain what he meant. Once you understand his intent, start a more coherent version of his sentence and have him finish it. After the student has read the revision, ask him if it matches what he meant. If not, work on the sentence until the revision accurately expresses the student's original idea.

Problems with Content and Organization

Students often have difficulty finding enough to say in their writing assignments and organizing their thoughts in a logical or interesting manner. Suggest that they begin by making notes of everything they can think of pertaining to the topic. The next step is to select from their notes the specific points and details that they want to include in their composition. Then they should organize those points and details in the order in which they want to include them. They should do all of this *before* writing their first draft. After the first draft is written, they should read it to see if they want to add anything more or to rearrange any of the points.

A Summary of Do's and Don'ts

1. Do tailor writing assignments to meet the students' needs and capabilities.
2. Do make sure that students understand the purpose and value of writing practice.
3. Do have students keep an orderly composition book for all their writing.
4. Do make sure that written work is evaluated, and when appropriate, have students write at least a second draft.
5. Do provide opportunities for students to share their writing with each other.
6. Don't expect the students' writing levels to be as high as their reading levels.
7. Don't allow writing assignments to become more important than the lessons and other necessary reinforcement activities.

6. Using the Lesson Notes

Because you are already familiar with the principles and procedures that pertain to the lessons in general from reading the previous chapters in this manual, you have the necessary foundation for sound instructional practices. The lesson notes address some specific points for the individual lessons. As part of class preparation, you should review the notes for the lesson assigned for homework. You should also read the notes for the lesson which you will be previewing to decide on how best to introduce the reading and to note any suggestions and reminders that might be helpful to the students when they are doing their homework.

Keep in mind that the lesson notes are only suggestions based on the experience of other reading teachers. If you try one of the suggestions a few times and find it doesn't work, disregard it.

Items of Primary and Secondary Emphasis

In most cases, the items listed under the "Primary emphasis" heading deal with reading comprehension, forming and writing reasoned opinions, and vocabulary development and review. Reading comprehension always receives primary emphasis because students are applying what they are learning to all parts of the lesson. Sometimes, the first time a particular task is introduced as an exercise, it is listed under "Primary emphasis" also.

Items listed under "Secondary emphasis" receive less emphasis in the lesson. Many are skills which have been introduced previously and are now being reinforced. Occasionally, a task normally receiving secondary emphasis, such as learning common prefixes, is listed under "Primary emphasis" because more emphasis than usual has been given to a particular skill in order to review and assess the students' progress.

The Reading Selection

The lesson notes contain suggestions for introducing the reading selections and for discussing them. The reading segment of the lesson demands more flexibility on the teacher's part than any other. Students vary greatly in ability and motivation. Remember that the key to helping students make the greatest gains in the least amount of time is observation. Carefully monitoring your students' progress will help you to develop sound procedures for improving reading and comprehension skills.

Developing Your Own Notes

Develop the habit of keeping your own notes. Take time at the end of each class session to write down any remarks or reminders about particular difficulties students may have had with the lesson. Also make note of specific words or skills for which you may want to develop reinforcement activities.

Also, be sure to keep notes of any procedures and techniques which seem to work well. Often you will hit upon an excellent way to present a certain skill or concept. Take some time to jot down your idea, especially if you know that you won't have the opportunity to use it again until a much later time. So much patience and concentration is called for in teaching reading that it's easy to forget those great ideas.

7. Lesson Notes for Book 8

Lesson 1
Houdini: His Legend and His Magic

Primary emphasis

- Reading comprehension (biography)
- Forming a reasoned opinion
- Vocabulary development (synonyms)
- Putting statements in proper sequence

Secondary emphasis

- Using context clues
- Using the dictionary
- Learning word origins

Words for Study

The Words for Study section includes words that appear in this lesson which have not appeared previously in this controlled-vocabulary series. As was the case with the preceding books in this series, most of the new words appear in subsequent reading selections and exercises so that students have many opportunities to work with them. Thus, there is no need to strive for immediate mastery; mastery will come with practice.

It is recommended that the words be pronounced and briefly discussed prior to the students' completing the reading independently. If done in a brief and informal manner, this practice increases students' confidence in their ability to complete the lesson. Also, it often arouses their curiosity about the reading.

Not all words need to be defined during this brief discussion. For example, if a student asks what the word *shackles* means, tell him that the word will appear in the lesson and that the context in which it appears will help him to understand the meaning of the word. If necessary, review the meaning of *context*.

Times occur, however, when it is helpful to give an on-the-spot definition, sentence, or example of an unfamiliar word. Perhaps a student needs to know that he has a working relationship with you. Perhaps he has had a difficult day and needs a few moments to center himself on the work. Whatever the reason, a few seconds of friendly conversation is more important than reminding him of the value of context clues.

The Words for Study section provides an excellent resource for spelling quizzes, brief writing assignments, and classroom games. Suggestions regarding these activities are found in Chapter 4 of this manual.

The Reading Selection

Tell students that all the readings in Book 8 have been taken from the works of professional writers.

Knowing this fact has proved to be an excellent source of motivation for many students.

Introduce this reading selection by pointing out that it was taken from *Houdini: His Legend and His Magic* by Doug Henning. It is helpful to have this book available for students to peruse because it has many illustrations. Review the meaning of the term *biography*. Because some students have difficulty distinguishing between nonfiction and fiction, it may be helpful to review these terms, also.

Generally, all initial readings of the selections should be done for homework. However, because this is the first lesson, allot time for an oral first reading in class. This gives you an opportunity to assess the strengths and weaknesses of students' oral reading abilities. Begin by reading the first part of the story yourself, and then ask for volunteers to continue.

Good oral reading skills often foster not only more proficient reading but also a greater appreciation of reading. Oral reading practice is especially welcomed by adults who would like to read with more confidence to their children or, occasionally, to their peers.

After reading the selection aloud, discuss it in a general way. This gives students a chance to get a sense of the selection as a whole while giving you the opportunity to assess their comprehension skills. Because the comprehension exercises often address specific reading skills, the general discussion can be focused on personal thoughts about or reactions to the reading. Otherwise, students are likely to develop the habit of thinking that reading comprehension merely consists of recalling as much as you can about what you have read and nothing more.

When you have completed the general discussion of the reading selection, preview the exercises to be done for homework. Since this is the first lesson, take plenty of time and be sure all students understand how to do each exercise. If necessary, have students complete an item in each exercise so that they have a thorough understanding of how to do the work.

During the homework review, allot some time to help students analyze the dictionary entry for *Houdini*. Have them look up the entry for *Houdini* in a current dictionary. Briefly discuss the entry formats and remind students that they will find the dictionary an excellent resource in completing many of the exercises in *Challenger 8*.

Exercise 1: Understanding the Reading

During the homework preview, remind students that they are to refer to the story for any answer they cannot recall. If students seem to think that having to go back to the story for an answer is a sign of poor reading, tell them that this simply isn't so. If anything, it is a sign of good scholarship.

Tell students to complete *all* the questions for this and all other exercises in Book 8. If you establish this pattern of completing all the work at the outset, students will more quickly develop a habit of thoroughness about their work.

Some students have the misconception that they should skip a question if they are not completely certain that their answer is correct. Remind these students that a blank is marked as an incorrect answer on many tests and that these questions give them an opportunity to practice the art of "intelligent guessing."

A score of 80% or better should be considered good on comprehension questions of this type. During the homework review, help students who had difficulty with the last three questions to find clues in the reading which indicate the correct answer. Students often need to be reminded that having some understanding of the author's motives or attitude is a valuable reading skill because it helps them to form a more reasoned judgment of what they read.

Exercise 2: What Do You Think?

During the homework preview, encourage students to write well-developed answers for these questions. Point out that the directions require them to support their thoughts and opinions with sound reasons.

When going over this section with the students during the homework review, make sure the answers are written in complete sentences. Initially, students may have difficulty putting their answers in sentence form, but with practice they will become increasingly proficient.

Also, help students make any necessary spelling and grammatical corrections. It may be helpful to remind them that writing is a form of communication, and spelling and grammar rules have been designed to make this communication clearer. When students begin to see that their writing improves with this attention to corrections and that there is no penalty for having made an error in the first place, they tend to progress more rapidly.

Exercise 3: Synonyms

During the homework preview, suggest that students use the process of elimination and a dictionary to complete this exercise. Review the process of elimination if students are unsure of what you mean. This is a useful tool that will help students complete many of the exercises in this book. During the homework review, review the meaning of *synonym*. Again, 80% or better should be considered a good score for exercises of this type.

Exercise 4: Names That Have Made the Dictionary

During the homework preview, point out that in addition to correct spellings and word definitions, dictionaries contain other interesting information, including the origins of many words. Students may not be aware that people's names are one source of words in our language. During the review you might ask if students know any other words that come from people's names. *Boycott*, *cardigan*, *dunce*, *Pullman*, *valentine*, and *silhouette* are some other examples.

Exercise 5: Challenges

During the homework preview, point out that there may be more than one possible way to order these sets of sentences. Students are asked to put them into a *sensible* order.

During the homework review, you may wish to have students act out these challenges in class. They can then see if the order they selected is a sensible one.

Note

After students have gone over the exercises and made any necessary corrections during the homework review, give them an opportunity to ask questions or make comments about what they have just accomplished. Students who are not familiar with the format of *Challenger* workbooks may feel overwhelmed by the work. Point out strengths they have shown in completing the work. Remind them that this is only the first lesson and that they will get used to the work more quickly than they think possible.

Lesson 2
Mirror, Mirror, on the Wall...

Primary emphasis
- Reading comprehension (nonfiction)
- Forming a reasoned opinion
- Comparing points of view
- Reading a map

Secondary emphasis
- Vocabulary development (antonyms)
- The suffix -*logy*
- Using the dictionary

The Reading Selection

During the homework preview, read aloud the two paragraphs which introduce this selection and briefly discuss students' views on the use of cosmetics and the concepts *primitive* and *civilized*.

During the homework review, discuss the author's thoughts about our use of the words *primitive* and *civilized*. One activity that has helped students to understand the author's point more clearly is to make two columns marked *primitive* and *civilized* on the chalkboard. Then have the students list words we use to label people and record them in the appropriate column. For example, they may list *simple* for primitive people and *sophisticated* for civilized people. Students also find it helpful to explore questions such as "What is the difference between our use of these terms and that of an anthropologist?" and "Is one use better than another?"

Because the theme of Unit 1 is appearances, another discussion topic or writing activity is to have students more fully explore the author's view that cosmetics are related to our sense of personal identity. This concept can be extended to include clothing styles and jewelry as well. Suggested questions include "What are we trying to tell others by the way we dress?" and "Does this message reveal our true selves?"

Exercise 1: Understanding the Reading

Remind students to read the selection carefully *prior* to answering the comprehension questions. Not only will their reading improve, but also they will find *Challenger 8* far more enjoyable.

The answer to question 1 cannot be found in the reading selection. Mention this during the homework preview and tell students to make an "intelligent guess."

Exercise 2: More about *We* and *They*

During the homework preview, have the students study the directions and examples carefully. Be sure they understand what is expected of them. Many students have the tendency to skim directions, skip examples, and then wonder why a particular section of work is so confusing.

During the review, give students a chance to discuss and debate any differences they may have in their responses to the situations in question 1. Follow this up with discussions of questions 2 and 3.

Exercise 3: Antonyms

During the homework preview, remind students to use a dictionary and the process of elimination to complete this exercise. Review the terms *synonym* and *antonym* during the homework review.

Exercise 4: The Suffix *-logy*

Students should also use the process of elimination and a dictionary to complete this exercise. They need not complete the exercise in order but should be encouraged to start with what they consider the easiest items. It may be helpful to review the pronunciation of the words in the column on the left. In this type of exercise, students should strive to have all answers correct—including the spelling.

Exercise 5: More about Melanesia

During the homework preview, have students find Melanesia on a globe or map of the world. This will give them a better sense of the location and size of Melanesia. Most students have no idea that this part of the world even exists.

It is helpful to have pictures of Melanesian life available during the homework review. You might also discuss the function of the international date line, since the theme of Unit 2 is time.

Lesson 3
Television: The Image-Maker

Primary emphasis
- Reading comprehension (nonfiction)
- Forming a reasoned opinion
- Interpreting a cartoon
- Vocabulary (synonyms and antonyms)

Secondary emphasis
- The suffix *-ist*
- Using context clues
- Completing a puzzle (anagrams)

The Reading Selection

Introduce this selection by reading the introductory paragraph aloud and asking students to predict what the author will say. During the general discussion of the article, allow students to react to Mr. Mander's opinions. This article presents an excellent opportunity to discuss the difference between fact and opinion. Have students select specific statements from the article and decide as a group whether they are statements of fact or opinion.

A suggested composition assignment to follow up this reading is "When I Imitated Television Behavior." An activity that some students have found enlightening is to make a commitment to forego all television for a week and then to discuss the results.

Exercise 2: More on the Media

During the homework preview, briefly discuss some of the ways in which cartoonists express their opinions. During the review, allow ample time for students to share their answers to questions 2 and 3.

As a follow-up activity, students might bring in cartoons from the editorial page of a newspaper or from a magazine and discuss how the cartoonists make their points.

Exercise 3: Synonyms and Antonyms

Remind students to use a dictionary if necessary to complete this exercise.

Exercise 4: the Suffix *-ist*

If you sense students will have difficulty with this exercise, complete the first item with them during the preview. After they have read the first sentence, ask them to identify what they consider a key word. Most students will respond *trance*. Then, ask them to locate the word in the left column which they associate with *trance*. Generally, they have no trouble finding the correct answer, and they better understand how to complete the exercise. Mention that this is an example of using context clues, a valuable reading skill, and review the meaning of *context*.

Review the pronunciation of the words in the column at the left during the homework review.

Exercise 5: A Familiar Television Phrase

Students may have difficulty getting started with this puzzle. You may want to help them complete a few of the items during the homework preview.

Tell students to skip around, to skim, and to use the sums as clues. For example, most students know that the answer for clue 4 is *never*. Ask them what letter of this word is least used. Their response is usually *v*, which is correct. Tell them to skim the puzzle for a word with a *v*. They will spot *nerve* and *drove* and can quickly see that the correct space is *nerve*. Remind them that the *n* is to be written on the fourth blank below the clues because it is the fourth clue. If they fill in the blanks for the television phrase as they go along, they may guess the answer before the puzzle is finished. This, in turn, will give them the initial letters of the remaining words.

Also, point out to them that the clue numbers always add up to 65, both horizontally and vertically. This may help them to find the right answers and also to know whether or not they have the right answers.

Lesson 4
Keeping up with the Joneses

Primary emphasis
- Reading comprehension (nonfiction)
- Forming a reasoned opinion
- Analogies

Secondary emphasis
- The suffix *-ism*
- Using context clues
- Spelling

The Reading Selection

This selection is not easy to read or to comprehend. In introducing it, you might mention that Veblen's book is required reading for many college courses. You may wish to consider having the students read and discuss the selection in class rather than assigning it for homework. Or you may decide to review their answers to Exercise 1 prior to the general discussion to make sure they have understood the basic points. During the general discussion, allow time for students to discuss their reactions to the points Veblen raises.

As a follow-up composition topic, students might describe a time when they bought something simply because someone else had one or because they wanted to impress someone else.

Exercise 2: What Do You Think?

For question 3, suggest that students phrase their objections in the form of quoted statements. For example, a student may list his tape deck as the first item and write "I can't concentrate or fall asleep at night unless my favorite tape is playing."

A discussion topic that students have found interesting is whether or not consumerism is the problem that Veblen suggests it is. Encourage students to relate the theme of appearances to consumerism, if possible (because this type of discussion can turn into a heated debate in spite of your best efforts).

Exercise 3: Word Relationships

Students often have difficulty with this type of exercise. Help them get started by going over the first question during the preview. Ask them to explain the relationship between *Houdini* and *illusionist*. Then have them read the four choices and decide which pair of words expresses a similar relationship. Most students will have no trouble selecting *Edison is to genius*.

Remind students that the process of elimination is often helpful in selecting the correct answer, and that they may use the dictionary to look up unfamiliar words. Whether or not you choose to introduce the term *analogy* is up to you. Some students are impressed by this word.

Exercise 4: The Suffix *-ism*

During the preview, remind students that the process of elimination and context clues are helpful tools in completing this type of exercise.

Review the meanings of the suffixes *-logy, -ist,* and *-ism* during the homework review.

Exercise 5: Spelling Check

During the preview, draw students' attention to the fact that in some sentences all the words may be spelled correctly. During the review, you may want to discuss the meaning of *et cetera*. Make sure *Bulletin* in number 8 is capitalized.

Lesson 5
While the Auto Waits

Primary emphasis
- Comprehension of literature (short story)
- Forming a reasoned opinion
- Vocabulary review
  1. Which word does not fit?
  2. Word associations

Secondary emphasis
- Review of suffixes
- Using context clues

The Story

During the homework preview, mention that, unlike the readings in the previous lessons, this is a work of fiction. Review the meanings of *fiction* and *nonfiction*. To introduce the story you might mention that O. Henry is known for his surprise endings. Students who have used earlier books in the *Challenger* series are familiar with O. Henry's work.

As an additional writing activity, the students can briefly summarize the theme of appearances as it relates to the five different readings.

Exercise 1: Understanding the Story

The answers to several of these questions are not specifically given in the reading selection but can be inferred from the information given. If students have trouble drawing the correct conclusions, discuss the process of inferring the best choice.

Exercise 2: What Do You Think?

During the review, discuss the concept of pretenses and its relationship to the theme of appearances.

Exercise 3: Which Word Does Not Fit?

Remind students that a dictionary and the process of elimination will be helpful in completing this exercise.

Exercise 4: More about O. Henry

During the homework preview, tell students to read each entire sentence before attempting to find the correct response. Tell them to pay attention to word endings and context clues in deciding which word to place in each blank.

When students have finished filling in the blanks, have them read the entire exercise again for comprehension.

Review the various suffixes in the groups of words on the left during the homework review.

Exercise 5: Pretenses in the Park

During the homework preview, have students study the example. Stress that they are to match the people listed above with statements they would make if they were *pretending*. Therefore, they are to look for the opposite of what the people would say if they were telling the truth.

As a follow-up activity, students enjoy selecting their own "people" words (such as bookworm, gadabout, homebody, hypocrite, and scatterbrain) and creating their own bits of pretentious dialogue to go with them.

Review: Lessons 1-5

It should be emphasized to the students that this is a review, not a test. These exercises are opportunities to review words and concepts that have been introduced in previous lessons. Material is often presented in new ways to both challenge the students and to arouse their interest. Preview each exercise included in the review as you do in other lessons. An overall score of 80% or better on the review should be considered excellent.

Exercise 2: Word Review

Remind students to read the entire statement before selecting the correct response. Both context clues and the process of elimination are helpful tools.

Exercise 3: Synonyms and Antonyms

Many students find this exercise more manageable if they first complete all the synonyms and then complete the antonyms.

Exercise 4: Faraway Places

An encyclopedia is recommended for this exercise, although most of the answers may be found in a good dictionary. You may want to have students complete this exercise during class time if they don't have access to other references outside of class.

Exercise 5: A Final Word on Appearances

During the homework preview, begin reading the poem aloud to the class. After two or three stanzas, ask for volunteers to continue the reading. Expression, especially the blind men's observations, should be encouraged.

After discussing students' responses to the comprehension questions, discuss the relationship of this poem to the theme of Unit 1, appearances.

You may wish to assign a composition to bring this unit of work to a conclusion. Here are some suggestions for composition topics relating to the theme of appearances.

1. When I Was Deceived by Appearances
2. Why I Think It Is (or Isn't) Okay to Create an Illusion
3. When I Pretended to Be What I Wasn't
4. Why I Think It Is (or Isn't) Okay to Watch Television
5. Television Has (or Doesn't Have) Too Much Influence in Our Lives
6. I Prefer Reality to Illusions (or I Prefer Illusions to Reality) Because...

Lesson 6
Time

Primary emphasis
- Reading comprehension (nonfiction)
- Forming a reasoned opinion
- Using context clues

Secondary emphasis
- Reviewing common prefixes
- Learning word origins
- Interpreting a diagram

Words for Study
During the homework preview, discuss any of the Words for Study that are not familiar to the students and relate them to the Unit 2 theme, Time.

The Reading Selection
Introduce this selection by briefly discussing what students think of when they hear the word *time*. Make a list of their responses for later reference. During the general discussion, you may want students to note which of their responses were mentioned in the reading. Discuss the authors' contention that *time* cannot be defined. Have students look up the entries for *time* in an unabridged dictionary and discuss whether or not they think *time* is adequately defined.

Exercise 1: Understanding the Reading
Review the process of inferring answers from the reading and of "intelligent guessing" during the homework preview.

Exercise 2: What Do You Think?
Encourage the students to personalize their answers. For example, "I save time when I wash the dishes right after eating. When I let them pile up, they are harder to clean."

Suggested follow-up composition topics for this exercise are: "I Never Have Enough Time to . . . " and "How I Like to Spend My Time."

Exercise 3: Durations
Students will need "intelligent guessing," the process of elimination, and context clues to complete this exercise. Encourage them to use the dictionary for unfamiliar words. Review the meaning of *durations* during the homework review.

Exercise 4: Origins of Calendar Words
During the preview, remind students to read each entire sentence before deciding on the correct response. Remind them to read the entire exercise through for comprehension after they have filled in all the blanks.

Review the meaning of the term *prefix* during the homework review. Then review the meanings of the prefixes used in this exercise.

Exercise 5: The Flower Clock
During the preview, make sure students understand the concept of the flower clock and can read and interpret the diagram. The time that particular flowers open and close will vary, depending upon such factors as latitude and climate.

Lesson 7
Once upon a Time...

Primary emphasis
- Reading comprehension (nonfiction)
- Using context clues
- Interpreting a chart

Secondary emphasis
- Vocabulary (scientific terms)
- Putting events in proper sequence
- Singular and plural nouns

Words for Study
It is helpful to discuss briefly the meanings of difficult words during the preview.

The Reading Selection
Most people have heard something about dinosaurs. Tell students that this reading describes how scientists have learned about these huge, extinct animals. It is helpful to have pictures or toy models of several different types of dinosaurs for students to look at.

As a follow-up activity, some students may want to find out more about the different types of dinosaurs or about other extinct animals and prepare a written or oral report for the class. You can suggest resources that interested students might use.

Exercise 1: Understanding the Reading
After questions 8 and 9 have been discussed during the homework review, make sure that students understand the difference between *theory* and *fact*.

Exercise 2: Scientific Classification: Part 1
During the homework preview, direct students' attention to the chart in Exercise 3 and tell them that it may also help them to complete Exercise 2. Remind students to read the entire exercise through for comprehension after they have filled in all the blanks.

Exercise 3: Scientific Classification: Part 2

During the preview, make sure students can read and interpret the chart. During the homework review, briefly discuss the reason for the use of Latin and Greek in scientific classifications.

Exercise 4: Putting Events in Order

After the correct sequence has been established during the homework review, have students read all three paragraphs aloud for comprehension. Ask students why they think so many fossils were preserved at this particular site.

Exercise 5: A Review of Singular and Plural Words

Some students are unaware of the fact that plural forms of words are cited in dictionaries. It may be helpful to complete one or two items during the homework preview so that they know how to find this information. If the dictionary gives two plural forms, remind students to list both.

Lesson 8
How to Live to Be 100 or More

Primary emphasis
- Reading comprehension (autobiographical humor)
- Forming a reasoned opinion
- Vocabulary review
- Learning common prefixes

Secondary emphasis
- Interpreting sayings
- Using the dictionary
- Solving a puzzle (cryptogram)

The Reading Selection

It is helpful to have pictures of George Burns available when introducing this selection. Most students will recognize him. Many of them have seen George Burns in movies or on television. A suggested follow-up activity is to have students read the excerpt aloud imitating George Burns's style.

A follow-up composition topic that students have enjoyed is "Why I Want (or Don't Want) to Live to Be 100."

Exercise 1: Understanding the Reading

Analyzing humor is not easy. It is often difficult to tell why a particular incident is amusing. If you think your students may have difficulty answering question 1, you might briefly discuss a well-known comedian's style and ask them to explain why they think it is funny.

Exercise 2: More Old and Not-So-Old Sayings

During the homework review, discuss the meanings of any of the sayings which students don't understand.

Exercise 4: More Common Prefixes

After going over the answers, review the meanings of the prefixes in this exercise.

Exercise 5: Can You Crack the Code?

If students seem bewildered by this puzzle, have a United States map available during the preview to help them figure out the outlined state. This will give them seven more letters. If they are still confused, have them put C's above all the D's in the puzzle and A's above all the P's. They should then be able to complete it on their own.

Lesson 9
What Will the Future Bring?

Primary emphasis
- Reading comprehension (nonfiction)
- Forming a reasoned opinion
- Analogies
- Interpreting poetry

Secondary emphasis
- Learning common prefixes
- Using context clues

The Reading Selection

During the preview, introduce the selection by discussing any unfamiliar words in the Words for Study section and by reading the introductory paragraph. Ask students if they ever read the astrology column in the newspaper or if they have tried any other methods to tell what might happen in the future.

After having discussed the reading during the homework review, many students like to act out the assassination scene in William Shakespeare's *Julius Caesar*. Another follow-up activity that has proved enjoyable is to have students research and bring in additional material on Nostradamus or Merlin.

Exercise 1: Understanding the Reading

Make sure students understand the directions for this exercise. Some students will tend to write too general a description which bears no specific relationship to the theme of the future. During the homework review, discuss the excerpt from Schiller's poem to make sure students understand Schiller's point.

Exercise 2: What Do You Think?

A follow-up composition topic which builds on students' responses to this exercise is "What I Hope the Future Will Bring."

Exercise 3: Word Relationships

Remind students to first recognize the relationship between the given words and then to use the process of elimination to find a similar relationship among the answer choices.

Exercise 4: Still More Prefixes

Some students think that if they know the meaning of a prefix, they should automatically know the meaning of the word. Remind them that it doesn't always work this way and to use a dictionary if necessary. During the review, after going over the students' responses, review the meanings of these prefixes and the ones in Lesson 8.

Exercise 5: A Look Back

Read the poem aloud during the homework preview and have students read the poem aloud during the review. Discuss with the students changes that have occurred in our language since Shakespeare's time. For example, how would a contemporary writer or speaker say "ways be foul," "doth," and "keel the pot"?

Lesson 10
All Summer in a Day

Primary emphasis
- Comprehension of literature (short story)
- Forming a reasoned opinion
- Vocabulary review (synonyms)
- Reading and designing bar graphs

Secondary emphasis
- Using context clues
- Review of prefixes and suffixes

Words for Study

A brief discussion of difficult words during the preview is recommended.

The Story

Introduce the story by telling students that it is science fiction and asking if they can give any examples of science fiction that they are familiar with. Even if they have never read any science fiction, most people have seen one or more of the well-known movies of this genre, such as the *Star Wars* trilogy or *E.T.* Briefly discuss some of the qualities that make science fiction different from other forms of fiction.

As a follow-up writing activity, students may enjoy writing their own science fiction stories. Encourage them to give free rein to their imaginations. If they are willing, have them read their stories aloud to the class.

Exercise 1: Understanding the Story

For question 1, remind students that the term *setting* refers to both time and place.

Exercise 2: What Do You Think?

Question 2 can be the basis for an interesting follow-up discussion topic: "Will people be different in the future?" Related to this question is another suggested by Exercise 4: "Were people really different in the past?"

Exercise 4: Looking Backward

Review the meanings of the various prefixes, suffixes, and roots in the groups of words on the left.

As a follow-up activity to this exercise, you or your students could try to locate and bring to class some newspapers from years ago. They can then discuss various changes that have taken place in areas such as newspaper format, editorial views, photos and illustrations, advertisements, and so forth.

Exercise 5: The Days of Our Lives

During the homework preview, make sure students understand how to read and construct a bar graph. Point out that in Part A they should write a question mark if there is insufficient information on the graph to answer the question.

Review: Lessons 1-10

As with the review for Unit 1, remind students that this is not a test. These exercises are additional opportunities to review words and concepts that were introduced in previous lessons. Encourage students to refer to those lessons or to a dictionary for words they cannot recall. An overall score of 80% or better on a review exercise should be considered excellent.

Exercise 4: More Durations

Make sure students understand how to do this exercise during the homework preview. Go over the one that has been done, and have them complete the first sentence in class, if necessary. Remind them that context clues will be very helpful in determining which three prefixes to select from each group.

Exercise 5: Past, Present, and Future

Students who have worked in previous books in the *Challenger* series are familiar with this type of puzzle. Remind them to fill in the appropriate blanks for the quote as they answer each item. In this way, they can work back and forth between the clues and the quote, using context clues in the quote to complete partially filled-in words.

During the homework review, you may want to have students summarize the theme for Unit 2, Time, as it relates to the readings in these five lessons.

If you wish to assign a composition to conclude this unit of work, here are some suggestions for composition topics relating to the theme of time:

1. I Wish I Had Lived When...
2. If I Could Predict the Future I Would...
3. When I Wanted Time to Stand Still
4. When I Wanted Time to Fly
5. I Wish I Could Live 100 Years from Now Because...
6. When I Had the Time of My Life

Lesson 11
A Fable for Tomorrow

Primary emphasis
- Reading comprehension (nonfiction)
- Forming a reasoned opinion
- Reading a map and bar graph

Secondary emphasis
- Using context clues
- Learning word origins
- Using the dictionary

The Reading Selection

This reading introduces the theme for Unit 3, the Good Earth. Introduce the reading by explaining that it is comprised of two excerpts from different sources. Mention that the first part of the reading is taken from Rachel Carson's well-known book *Silent Spring* and that the second excerpt is about Rachel Carson herself. Review the terms *fable* and *biography*.

A follow-up discussion is recommended on the topic of substances and practices that are currently considered harmful to the environment. You may want to develop a class or group project throughout this unit by having students collect items from newspapers, magazines, and other sources that pertain to environmental pollution and protection issues. Students could create classroom or bulletin board displays, or a scrapbook with the materials they gather. Groups of students might give presentations on specific issues when the unit comes to an end.

Exercise 2: What Do You Think?

Have Chief Seattle's statement read aloud during the homework preview and briefly discuss what it means. Allow time during the homework review for a general discussion of students' reactions to the questions and to the statement.

Exercise 3: What Is the Nobel Prize?

During the preview, remind students to read the entire exercise through for comprehension after they have filled in all the blanks. Like DDT, dynamite has proved to be a mixed blessing. Although it is not included in the exercise, you may wish to mention that Nobel was despondent over the consequences of his invention.

Exercise 4: Names in Nature

Encourage students to use a dictionary in completing this exercise, but warn them that not all references agree on the origins of all words. Etymology is an inexact science, and some dictionaries may differ about the origins of the words included in this exercise. For some words, there may be no source given in the dictionary. Remind students to use the process of elimination if they have doubts about which answer choice is best. Review the term *etymology* during the homework review and discuss various ways that words enter our language.

Exercise 5: The Good Earth

During the preview, tell students that they will need to study both the map and the bar graph in order to answer the questions which follow. Point out that in Part A they should write a question mark if there is insufficient information on the graph to answer the question. In Part B, however, they are also to use their own background information to decide whether or not the conclusions are reasonable. Discrepancies among students' answers may be the result of differing background knowledge. Allow time during the review to discuss any statements where there are differing responses.

Lesson 12
Life on Earth

Primary emphasis
- Reading comprehension (nonfiction)
- Forming a reasoned opinion
- Vocabulary (synonyms and antonyms)

Secondary emphasis
- Charting information
- Using reference materials
- Solving a puzzle (spelling check)

Words for Study

This list is both longer and more difficult than most of the Words for Study lists. Briefly discuss the meanings of the more difficult words during the homework preview. Use these words and concepts to introduce the reading selection.

The Reading Selection

During the general discussion of the reading selection, you might remind students of the fable by Rachel Carson in the previous lesson, and ask them how the concepts in this reading relate to Ms. Carson's ideas. Discuss what impact the rapid increase in human population has had on the other forms of life on the Earth.

If your students have begun a class project on environmental issues, have them look specifically for materials on ecology and the population explosion. If there is a current local environmental issue, such as a movement to clean up a polluted river or lake, or the location of a trash-burning plant, or the disposal of toxic wastes, you might invite one or two people who are knowledgeable about the details to discuss or debate the issue in your class.

Exercise 2: Understanding the Reading: Part 2

During the review, allow time for students to share their views on the "What do you think?" question. Have students define what is meant by a "successful" species. During the discussion you may want to make a list of things we are doing to "adapt our behavior to...our natural environment." Then you might generate a list of things we could do that are not yet generally being done. As a follow-up composition topic, students could write about "What We Can Do to Improve Our Natural Environment."

Exercise 4: Charting Information

A good dictionary will indicate what most but not all of the animals listed feed upon. In some cases, students may have to look up the meaning of a word in the dictionary definition of the animal to discover the proper category. For example, a dictionary says the vulture lives on "carrion." A student may have to look up *carrion* to determine in which category *vulture* belongs. An encyclopedia may be needed for those animals whose eating habits are not mentioned in the dictionary.

As a reinforcement activity, students working in pairs can develop other lists of animals, exchange lists, and research the eating habits of those animals.

Exercise 5: Spelling Check

Students not familiar with this type of puzzle may need to complete an answer or two during the homework preview. Remind students to check off the syllables as they use them. They need not work in the order in which the clues appear. Make sure students capitalize the answer to number 12.

Lesson 13
The Good Earth: Two Points of View

Primary emphasis
- Reading comprehension (nonfiction)
- Forming a reasoned opinion
- Interpreting a cartoon
- Using context clues
- Comparing and contrasting points of view

Secondary emphasis
- Word families
- Using reference materials
- Solving a puzzle (cryptogram)

The Reading Selection

Introduce this selection by having students read the three introductory paragraphs aloud during the homework preview. Find the Cascade Range on a map of the United States. (It extends from northern California, through Oregon and Washington, into British Columbia. Both Mount Rainier and Mount Saint Helens are in this range.)

Perhaps the most startling piece of information in this selection is the fact that it took ten million tons of rock to make a hundred thousand tons of copper which, in turn, is the amount of copper used to wire a city the size of Kansas City. You may want to have students try to estimate how much rock and copper are required to provide electrical wiring for the major cities in your state, using recent population figures as the basis for comparison with Kansas City.

Exercise 1: Understanding the Reading

Allow time during the review for students to exchange their views about the uses of natural resources. Students can continue their work on a class project by collecting information on the use and misuse of natural resources.

Exercise 2: The Earth: A Cartoonist's Point of View

Students with artistic ability may want to try drawing other cartoons that illustrate different aspects of environmental problems. A suggested follow-up discussion or composition topic is "What Are We Going to Do with All Our Trash?"

Exercise 3: Word Families

It is helpful to review the meanings of the words in the left column during the homework review and to discuss the meanings of the various prefixes and suffixes.

Exercise 4: America's Resources

Many students are unfamiliar with many of the places mentioned in this exercise. Remind them to use key words in the sentences as their guides for finding the correct answers. During the homework review, locate the various places on a map of the United States. Pictures also enable students to gain a better sense of these places.

Exercise 5: Can You Crack the Code?

Remind students that they did a similar puzzle in Lesson 8. If necessary, help them get off to a good start by having them put *C*'s above all the *A*'s. A dictionary or other reference work may be helpful for finding the names of the less familiar metals.

Lesson 14
Antaeus: Part I

Primary emphasis
- Comprehension of literature (short story)
- Forming a reasoned opinion
- Analogies

Secondary emphasis
- Compound words
- Using reference materials
- Vocabulary (mythological figures)

The Story

Inform students during the homework preview that "Antaeus" is a short story in two parts and that it will be concluded in Lesson 15. Tell them Antaeus is the name of a figure in Greek mythology but that this is a modern story. The meaning of the title will be discussed during the homework review.

Exercise 1: Understanding the Story

During the homework review, try to have a resource such as an encyclopedia or Bulfinch's *Mythology* available so that students can look up information on Antaeus. Ask them why they think Borden Deal titled his story "Antaeus."

Exercise 2: What Do You Think?

As a follow-up writing assignment or class discussion topic, ask students to predict what will happen in the next part of the story. Students working on class projects can collect information on national and worldwide farming problems.

Exercise 4: From the Earth

If students have trouble forming the names of the plants, tell them to use a dictionary to look up the words in List A. However, a dictionary will not give them all the information they need to complete this exercise. *The World Book Encyclopedia* is another good source for this information.

Lesson 15
Antaeus: Part II

Primary emphasis
- Comprehension of literature (short story)
- Forming a reasoned opinion
- Homonym review

Secondary emphasis
- Vocabulary (which word does not fit?)
- Solving a logic puzzle

Words for Study

Both the pronunciation and meanings of many of these words are difficult. Briefly discuss them during the homework preview.

Story

Since this story is in two parts, it is helpful to begin the general discussion by having students briefly summarize the entire story. Remind them of the predictions they made about what would happen in the second part of the story. Discuss how close they came to the real ending.

Exercise 2: What Do You Think?

During the preview, suggest that students might want to write their answers to question 1 in the form of a dialogue. After discussing students' responses to the two questions during the review, ask if they have any further ideas about why Borden Deal titled this story "Antaeus."

Exercise 3: Which Word Does Not Fit?

If students are confused by the five choices in number 1, remind them that Atlas was a Titan in Greek mythology, while the rest are Roman gods, and Atlas is also the only one for whom no planet is named.

Exercise 4: Homonym Review

During the preview, review the term *homonym*. Make sure students understand how to complete this exercise.

Exercise 5: Logic Problem

This is not an easy puzzle. During the homework preview, make sure students understand how to go about solving this logic problem. Go over the directions and the example carefully with them. If they still seem confused, you may want to have them fill in information from Clue 2 in class. Remind them to reread the clues as often as necessary to complete the puzzle. Be sure they understand that for each *Y* they fill in, they can add six *N*'s to the chart (three up and down and three across). Students will find it helpful if you mention that the key to the solution is using the process of elimination.

Review: Lessons 1-15

As with the previous reviews, remind students that this is not a test. These exercises are additional opportunities to review words and concepts that were introduced in previous lessons. Encourage students to refer to those lessons or to a dictionary for words they cannot recall. An overall score of 80% or better on a review exercise should be considered excellent.

Exercise 1: Definitions

Because much of the vocabulary in this unit has been difficult, you may want to develop one or more reinforcement activities to review words that are not included in this exercise or in Exercise 3. The Word Index for Lessons 11-15 at the back of this manual will help you select additional words.

Exercise 5: A Poet's Point of View

During the homework preview, read the poem aloud to the class. Give students the opportunity to read it aloud during the review. Have them take turns reading complete sentences. This practice helps students break the habit of thinking that a line of poetry is always a complete sentence. After discussing their responses to questions 1 and 2, give students an opportunity to share their responses to number 3.

Because this review concludes this unit on environmental issues, allow students time during the homework review to discuss their concern or, perhaps, their lack of concern for the environment. They should be finishing up their work on their class project. You may also want to make a written assignment based on any of the topics covered by their project. If your class did not participate in a class project, you may wish to conclude this unit of work with a composition relating to the theme, the Good Earth. Here are some topic suggestions:

1. I think (or don't think) pollution is a problem because...
2. I think man will (or will not) continue to be a "successful" species because...
3. I think the world's natural resources are (or are not) being poorly managed because...
4. At Times I Feel Close to Nature
5. The Most Urgent Environmental Problem

Lesson 16
Life without Furnace, Pipe, or Wire

Primary emphasis
- Reading comprehension (nonfiction)
- Forming a reasoned opinion
- Outlining
- Writing a well-developed paragraph

Secondary emphasis
- Using context clues
- Using reference materials

The Reading Selection

During the preview, tell students that the theme of this unit is Change. Introduce this reading by having the three introductory paragraphs read aloud. Ask students to name some things in their homes that would not have been found in nineteenth century homes. During the review, students might discuss our modern concepts of comfort, leisure time, and basic necessities in relation to the description of nineteenth century life in the reading. A suggested follow-up composition topic is "What I Would Miss the Most if I Had to Live in a Nineteenth Century House."

Exercise 1: Understanding the Reading

During the preview, discuss the value of outlining as a means of ordering information so that it can be better understood and remembered. Describe the process for students who are unfamiliar with building an outline. If students have trouble with this exercise, you may want to have them outline one or two more readings or short articles as reinforcement activities. Be sure to select readings or articles that have a logical, straightforward organization.

Exercise 2: What Do You Think?

Students often ask if they should answer these questions in terms of their own lives or of society in general. Encourage them to think in terms of society in general.

Exercise 3: Using Context Clues

Remind students to read each quotation through for comprehension after filling in the blanks.

Exercise 4: Writing about Change

Encourage students to make a brief outline of their thoughts about the quotation they select before writing their paragraph. This will help them to organize their thoughts and to decide which details to include in their paragraphs. It is most helpful to react to these paragraphs primarily on the basis of content, organization, and style.

Exercise 5: Inventors and Their Inventions

Many dictionaries note only that these men were inventors, so a reference work such as *The World Book Encyclopedia* is recommended for this exercise. If necessary, allow time for students to complete it in class.

Lesson 17
A Marriage Proposal

Primary emphasis
- Comprehension of literature (drama)
- Forming a reasoned opinion
- Predicting an ending
- Vocabulary
  1. Synonyms
  2. Monetary terms

Secondary emphasis
- Word families
- Using context clues
- Using the dictionary

The Play
In introducing this play, tell students that it is set in Russia toward the end of the last century. Help them to pronounce the Russian names. Have students act out the scene during the homework review. Encourage them to play the parts as broadly as they wish. If your students enjoy reading plays, you may want to bring in copies of this play and have students act out the entire play. It can be found in various anthologies.

Exercise 2: You Be the Playwright
Allow students to read aloud or act out as many of their responses as they wish. Then briefly discuss how close their endings came to the actual ending of the play (see the Answer Key for a brief summary).

Exercise 3: More about Anton Chekhov
Remind students to read the entire exercise through for comprehension after filling in all the blanks.

Exercise 5: Foreign Currency
If you or any of your students have examples of foreign coins or paper money, it is interesting to bring these to class for the others to see.

Lesson 18
The Significance of Change

Primary emphasis
- Reading comprehension (nonfiction)
- Forming a reasoned opinion
- Writing optimistic and pessimistic responses

Secondary emphasis
- Vocabulary
  1. Antonyms
  2. Word associations
- Solving a puzzle (anagrams)

The Reading Selection
This reading is excerpted from Leo Buscaglia's best-selling book *Love*. Students—especially young adults—have found this book helpful, and you may wish to have a few copies in the classroom for them to borrow.

During the general discussion of the reading, it is helpful to discuss the things which Buscaglia lists as being part of all learning: searching, finding, analyzing, evaluating, experiencing, accepting, rejecting, practice, and reinforcement. Ask your students if they agree that learning involves all of these activities. Have them try to think of personal experiences or examples for each activity. In a follow-up composition, students might write about the learning process in general, or they might select the most important or most difficult part of the process and explain their selection.

Exercise 2: Optimists and Pessimists
During the preview, discuss the example and the differences between optimistic and pessimistic thinking to be sure students understand how to do this exercise. Students enjoy reading their statements aloud during the homework review. They also enjoy discussing which were easier to write—the optimists' or the pessimists' statements.

Exercise 5: An Inventor's Advice
Remind students to fill in Franklin's words of advice as they go along and that the numbers will add up to 65 both horizontally and vertically.

Lesson 19
It's Good to Be Alive

Primary emphasis
- Reading comprehension (autobiography)
- Forming a reasoned opinion
- Interpreting poetry

Secondary emphasis
- Understanding and drawing a diagram
- Contrasting points of view
- Analogies

The Reading Selection
Introduce this selection by having the introductory paragraph read aloud. Review the term *autobiography*. Briefly discuss the game of baseball and the role of the catcher. Pictures of baseball diamonds, stadiums, or teams at play can add interest to the discussion. During the general discussion, have students read aloud the poem which ends the selection. Discuss how it relates to Roy Campanella's philosophy as expressed throughout the reading.

Exercise 2: What Do You Think?

During the preview, you might suggest to the students that they make a brief outline of their thoughts and supporting details or reasons before beginning to write their paragraphs. Again, it is best to respond to students' writing on the basis of content, organization, and style.

Exercise 3: The Invention of Baseball

This description of an early form of baseball is difficult to read and students often complain that it is too complicated. This is partly due to the out-of-date language and partly because it is difficult to write a description of a step-by-step process. As a follow-up activity, it is helpful to have students try their hand at this type of writing. Suggested topics include:

Changing a Flat Tire
How to Tie a Shoe
Playing a Video Game
Playing Basketball (or some other sport)
How to Prepare a Meal
Giving Directions to the Student's Home

Exercise 4: Change: Another Type of Response

During the preview, read the poem aloud to the class. Have students take turns reading complete sentences aloud during the review. Prior to discussing the questions comparing Roy Campanella and Flick Webb, you may wish to have the students discuss questions about the poem itself, such as:

● Why do you think the poet named his basketball player Flick Webb?
● Based on its name, what kind of street would you expect Pearl Avenue to be?
● Based on its description, what kind of street is Pearl Avenue?
● What is the parallel between Pearl Avenue and Flick Webb's life?

Lesson 20
Heir to Tradition

Primary emphasis

- Reading comprehension (nonfiction)
- Forming a reasoned opinion
- Interpreting poetry

Secondary emphasis

- Using references
- Vocabulary (synonyms and antonyms)
- Spelling

The Reading Selection

During the homework preview, make sure that students have a sense of what the title means. This will help them to better understand the ideas presented in the reading. These ideas may be difficult for students to comprehend. Allot enough time during the general discussion and the review of the comprehension questions to be sure that students grasp the fundamental points that Overstreet makes.

Exercise 2: Reacting to the Reading

As a follow-up activity to question 3, students might follow through on one or more of the ways to establish a link with the past that they have listed in their responses. For instance, if a student listed reading some of the classics, he could develop a reading list and give reasons for his selections. A student who listed visiting a museum could do so and give a report on his visit. Or someone who chose to talk with older people might interview an elderly person and write a report on the interview.

Exercise 3: A Poem by Langston Hughes

As before, read the poem aloud during the preview and give students the opportunity to read it aloud during the review. Have a globe or map of the world available so students can locate the various rivers. Discuss how this poem and the reading selection relate to the theme of this unit, Change.

Exercise 5: Spelling Check

Two of the incorrect words in this exercise are spelled correctly. Because of the context, however, the following are incorrect:

1. Sentence 5—*foul* should be *fowl*
2. Sentence 10—*forth* should be *fourth*

A suggested follow-up activity is to have students gather information about other holiday traditions to present to the class.

Review: Lessons 1-20

As with the previous reviews, this last review is not to be perceived as a test, but rather as a final opportunity to work with many of the words and concepts introduced in Book 8.

After any necessary corrections have been made by the students during the homework review, spend some time reviewing and evaluating the students' progress. In keeping with the theme of this unit, try to focus on the concept of change. Have students noticed a change in their reading ability? Have they experienced any changes in their thoughts about reading or about learning in general?

This is also an opportunity for you to share your perceptions. Needless to say, the emphasis should be placed on growth, for it is hoped that at least some of the readings in this workbook will have aroused the students' curiosity to learn more—to see that they are far more than "the powers and limitations they were born with" (Overstreet).

Answer Key for Book 8

Lesson 1

1 Understanding the Reading

1. b	3. b	5. a	7. a	9. d
2. c	4. b	6. b	8. d	10. a

2 What Do You Think?

1. Answers will vary. Accept any reasonable response.
2. Answers will vary. Accept any reasonable response.

3 Synonyms

1. display	6. amazing	11. overpower
2. confine	7. universal	12. hidden
3. burst	8. myth	13. dive
4. advertise	9. achievement	14. support
5. spellbound	10. disentangle	

4 Names That Have Made the Dictionary

1. braille, Braille
2. poinsettia, Poinsett
3. macintosh or mackintosh, Macintosh
4. Fahrenheit, Fahrenheit
5. lynch, Lynch
6. sandwich, Sandwich
7. derrick, Derick (or Derrick)
8. nicotine, Nicot

5 Challenges

1. 4, 3, 5, 2, 1
2. 5, 3, 4, 2, 1 or 5, 2, 3, 4, 1
3. 2, 5, 1, 3, 4 or 2, 5, 1, 4, 3

Lesson 2

1 Understanding the Reading

1. b	3. c	5. d	7. b
2. d	4. a	6. a	8. c

2 More about *We* and *They*

Answers will vary. Accept reasonable responses.

3 Antonyms

1. suddenly	6. dwindle	11. certainly
2. disfigure	7. frail	12. inflict
3. advanced	8. wastefulness	13. indifferent
4. fixed	9. jittery	14. dullness
5. careless	10. plain	

4 The Suffix *-logy*

1. zoology	5. ecology	9. sociology
2. meteorology	6. archaeology	10. theology
3. biology	7. pathology	11. etymology
4. psychology	8. geology	12. astrology

5 More about Melanesia

1. a	2. d	3. b	4. c	5. c

Lesson 3

1 Understanding the Reading

Answers will vary. Reasonable responses include:

1. The number of hours Americans watch TV each day indicates that television is a major influence in our lives.
2. Our image of the forest isn't the experience of being in the forest, but an edited version of it.
3. Some experiences keep recurring in your mind and you can't clear them out.
4. Images in the mind can affect the state of the body.
5. Many people's images or ideas are based on what they have seen on television.
6. People try to imitate the images they see on television and in the movies.
7. Many people use TV to learn how to handle problems in their lives.
8. Learning behavior from TV cannot substitute for experiencing real human relationships.

2 More on the Media

1. Joseph Farris seems to agree with Mr. Mander. Any of the following or similar details can be used as evidence: 99% of homes in the U.S. have TV sets; more than 80 million Americans watch TV on an average evening; the TV set is on more than six hours a day in the average household, and more than eight hours if there is a child; half of the average adult's nonsleeping, nonworking hours are spent watching TV.
2. Answers will vary. Accept any reasonable response.
3. Answers will vary.

3 Synonyms and Antonyms

1. antonyms	7. synonyms	13. antonyms
2. antonyms	8. antonyms	14. antonyms
3. synonyms	9. synonyms	15. synonyms
4. synonyms	10. synonyms	16. synonyms
5. antonyms	11. antonyms	
6. antonyms	12. synonyms	

4 The Suffix -ist

1. hypnotist
2. novelist
3. dramatist
4. journalist
5. activist
6. anthropologist
7. etymologist
8. archaeologist
9. alarmist
10. conformist
11. nonconformist
12. meteorologist

5 A Familiar Television Phrase

SHELF 12 FLESH	ROUTE 24 OUTER	SWEEP 6 WEEPS	POSES 20 POSSE	DAIRY 3 DIARY
NERVE 4 NEVER	DROVE 11 DOVER	ROGUE 25 ROUGE	SWING 8 WINGS	CRUEL 17 ULCER
TOWEL 16 OWLET	GROAN 5 ORGAN	ANGER 13 RANGE	KNEAD 22 NAKED	CANOE 9 OCEAN
ARISE 10 RAISE	NEWER 18 RENEW	MANES 2 NAMES	PEONS 14 OPENS	DOORS 21 ODORS
WORDS 23 SWORD	LATER 7 ALTER	NORSE 19 SNORE	SCARE 1 ACRES	AMPLE 15 MAPLE

The familiar television phrase: And now a word from our sponsor.

Lesson 4

1 Understanding the Reading

1. a   3. b   5. d   7. b   9. a
2. d   4. c   6. c   8. d   10. b

2 What Do You Think?

1. Answers will vary. Accept reasonable responses.
2. Answers will vary.
3. Answers will vary. Accept reasonable responses.

3 Word Relationships

1. b   3. c   5. a   7. a   9. c
2. c   4. d   6. c   8. c   10. b

4 The Suffix -ism

1. escapism
2. cynicism
3. individualism
4. heroism
5. terrorism
6. materialism
7. favoritism
8. capitalism
9. hypnotism
10. skepticism
11. idealism
12. patriotism

5 Spelling Check

1. origin
2. following
3. correct
4. etc.
5. humorous
6. correct
7. forty-two
8. Bulletin
9. cartoon
10. portraits

Lesson 5

1 Understanding the Story

1. b   3. c   5. d   7. b   9. c
2. a   4. d   6. c   8. a   10. c

2 What Do You Think?

1. Mr. Parkenstacker pretends to be a cashier in a restaurant. Answers will vary on why he does this. Accept reasonable responses.
2. Answers will vary.
3. Answers will vary.

3 Which Word Does Not Fit?

1. question
2. glaring
3. Sahara
4. hangman
5. idealistic
6. Montreal
7. fascination
8. self-seeking
9. nomad
10. stately
11. soar
12. unsuspecting
13. ballet
14. suggest
15. stillness
16. Wilhelmina

4 More about O. Henry

1. cleverly, scholarly, continually
2. originally, eventually, determinedly
3. necessity, majority, prosperity
4. objective, offensive, subjective
5. unbearable, valuable, unmistakable
6. confirmation, assumption, abbreviation
7. indication, limitation, quotation
8. cheerless, boundless, countless
9. bewilderment, fulfillment, bombardment
10. observation, relations, separation

5 Pretenses in the Park

1. wallflower
2. escapist
3. immigrant
4. skeptic
5. alarmist
6. Scrooge
7. manipulator
8. braggart
9. quibbler

Review: Lessons 1-5

1 Definitions

1. organism
2. luxury
3. leisure
4. trivia
5. status
6. prosperity
7. technique
8. neutrality
9. excerpt
10. assumption
11. feat
12. modesty
13. economy
14. illusion
15. fiction
16. penalty

2 Word Review

1. ecologist, glaring
2. executive, remarkably
3. immune, favoritism
4. Pierre, South Dakota
5. nonconformist, unbearable

6. minister, theology
7. accurately, entry
8. opposition, Nonetheless
9. Biology, organisms
10. ideal, instinct

3 Synonyms and Antonyms

1. plentiful, scarce
2. skepticism, conviction
3. imaginary, actual
4. cheerless, lighthearted
5. meekly, boastfully
6. reproduce, originate
7. confined, boundless
8. frill, necessity
9. modest, pretentious
10. upright, dishonorable
11. significant, uneventful
12. unbiased, subjective

4 Faraway Places

1. Guam
2. Vietnam
3. Budapest
4. Hawaii
5. Fiji
6. Sahara
7. Australia
8. Tahiti
9. New Guinea
10. Tasmania

5 A Final Word on Appearances

1. Each of the blind men thinks that the part of the elephant which he touches is representative of the whole.
2. There are differences of opinion among them about what an elephant is like. Each of them believes his opinion is right.
3. Answers will vary. Accept reasonable responses.
4. Answers will vary. Reasonable responses include: Appearances can be deceiving, especially if we are not open-minded. Knowing only partial facts can distort our perceptions of reality. We all tend to believe our opinions are correct and anyone who disagrees with us is wrong.

Lesson 6

1 Understanding the Reading

1. d	3. c	5. a	7. d	9. a
2. b	4. d	6. b	8. c	10. a

2 What Do You Think?

Answers will vary. Accept reasonable responses.

3 Durations

1. snowflake
2. Aspirin
3. Titanic
4. Chicago
5. whale
6. wrens
7. Philadelphia
8. Mayflower
9. Mercury
10. Pluto
11. fingernail
12. blood
13. gopher
14. tadpole, bullfrog
15. snail, senator
16. male, female
17. Easter

4 Origins of Calendar Words

1. inconsistent, indisputable, incomparable
2. represented, reinforced, readjusted
3. derived, denoted, desist
4. envisioned, encouraged, endorse
5. disorder, distant, disfigured
6. misgivings, misconception, misled
7. exceptional, exertions, exceptionally
8. unparalleled, unfortunate, ungodly

5 The Flower Clock

Answers will vary. Accept reasonable responses.

Lesson 7

1 Understanding the Reading

1. Most organisms get eaten soon after they die.
2. Any two of the following: It can be buried right after death in quicksand, bogs, swamps and stagnant water; it can be fossilized after drifting in rivers or lakes; it can be buried in sand or tar pits.
3. The tar pits of Rancho La Brea contain one of the world's richest fossil deposits. Fossils help us to understand what ancient animals were like.
4. An order is a category of animals or plants.
5. The Saurischia order is described in detail.
6. Accept four of the following or similar answers: Its legs were massive to support its incredible size. Its feet had short toes which spread to support its weight. There were elastic pads under the feet to keep it from getting stuck in soft ground. Some toes had claws to help it move in water and climb muddy banks. Its remarkable backbone was designed to support its huge weight. Its nostrils were high so it could breathe in the water without raising its head. Its long neck helped in gathering food.
7. Sauropods ate soft marsh plants, nipping them off with their blunt teeth. They were efficient food-gatherers with long necks that could reach far in all directions. Like modern reptiles, they probably needed only a fraction of the food a bird or mammal needs. They were different from most modern reptiles in that they ate plants, while most reptiles today are flesh eaters.

8. Two of the following: Flesh-eating dinosaurs ate all the others and then starved to death. This doesn't account for the death of dinosaurs living in the sea. A plague destroyed the dinosaurs. It is very rare for an entire species to be killed by a disease. An ice age caused the dinosaurs to disappear. There is no evidence of a sharp climate change at that time.

9. The Great Death of the dinosaurs was probably caused by a combination of factors rather than by a single event.

2 Scientific Classification: Part 1

1. method, arrange, related, indicates, relationships
2. scheme, judgment, specimens, agree, differ
3. words, scholars, common, correct, recognized
4. Seven, system, largest, two, plant
5. kingdom, divided, animals, backbones, phylum
6. characteristics, members, phylum, *Chordata*, class
7. class, milk, flesh, moles, insects
8. order, *Carnivora*, family, tails, *Felidae*
9. similar, different, breed, coyote, genus
10. basic, forms, one, two, genus

3 Scientific Classification: Part 2

1. d   2. b   3. c   4. d   5. b

4 Putting Events in Order

1. 4, 2, 3, 1, 5
2. 5, 1, 2, 4, 3
3. 4, 2, 1, 5, 3

5 A Review of Singular and Plural Words

1. appendixes, appendices
2. children
3. coyotes, coyote
4. crises
5. Englishmen
6. hippopotamuses, hippopotami
7. indexes, indices
8. knives
9. mice
10. phyla
11. radii, radiuses
12. sisters-in-law
13. series
14. shelves
15. species
16. studios
17. thieves
18. trout, trouts
19. vertebrae, vertebras
20. women

Lesson 8

1 Understanding the Reading

1. Answers may vary. Reasonable responses include:
   His Moses story: George Burns implies that he has been alive since the time of Moses. This exaggeration of his age makes the story funny.
   The story about his friend in Vancouver: People who walk for exercise usually walk a certain distance and then reverse directions and walk back to where they started. His friend walked five miles a day for six months—all in one direction.
   The story about his bypass surgery: He wasn't nervous about his surgery, but he found out later that his doctor had been a nervous wreck. George Burns, however, collapsed when he saw the doctor's bill.
2. "Laying an egg" is a slang expression for telling a joke that nobody laughs at. The college students didn't know who Betsy Ross was, so they didn't understand the joke George Burns told in his dressing room.
3. Life begins each day when you wake up. Accept reasonable answers for the second part of the question.
4. "Thinking young" involves thinking optimistically and having enthusiasm for what you do. People who "think young" lead full, vigorous lives. They keep active, make plans, meet people, and look to the future.

2 More Old and Not-So-Old Sayings

1. b   3. a   5. a   7. a
2. b   4. d   6. d

3 Vocabulary Review

Part A
1. trophies
2. birthday
3. Frigga
4. Swedish
5. primrose
6. ether
7. novel
8. mayor

Part B
1. perishable
2. intricate
3. uprooted
4. learned
5. wondrous
6. finite
7. pretentious
8. expressive

4 More Common Prefixes

1. a. abnormal
   b. absentee
   c. abduct
   d. abstain
   e. abstract
2. a. antiseptic
   b. antisocial
   c. antidote
   d. antimacassar
   e. antibiotic
3. a. foremost
   b. forebear
   c. foresight
   d. foretell
   e. forebode
4. a. postscript
   b. posterity
   c. posterior
   d. postmortem
   e. postpone
5. a. transform
   b. transgress
   c. transfix
   d. transplant
   e. transcribe

5 Can You Crack the Code?

Los Angeles, California

The four symbols on the Los Angeles seal represent the four governments in this city's history: Spain, Mexico, the California Republic, and the United States.

Lesson 9

1 Understanding the Reading

Reasonable responses include:

1. The Egyptians were among the earliest people to develop and use prophecy. Priests were trained to foretell the future of the Pharaohs and the nation.
2. He misinterpreted a prophecy by the oracle at Delphi and destroyed his own kingdom.
3. Jeremiah was one of the great Hebrew prophets in the Bible.
4. Also called the *Book of Changes*, the *I Ching* has been used by the Chinese people to foretell the future since the ninth century B.C.
5. Caesar ignored a seer's prophecy, "Beware the Ides of March," and was assassinated on that date.
6. They sacrificed bulls and men and, from the sounds of their victims' cries, they prophesied the future.
7. Merlin is a puzzling figure in British mythology who was a famous magician and prophet.
8. He was a French physician who prophesied in verses that were often puzzling, but many of which have proven accurate.
9. Currently a popular form of predicting the future, science fiction since World War II has dealt primarily with gloomy themes.
10. Schiller was a German poet who wrote that the future is inevitable and that sometimes future events can be foreseen.

2 What Do You Think?

Answers will vary. Accept reasonable responses.

3 Word Relationships

1. c	3. a	5. c	7. b	9. d
2. d	4. b	6. c	8. b	10. d

4 Still More Prefixes

1. concurred	5. emitted	9. submit
2. provoked	6. permissible	10. circumvent
3. adhere	7. superduper	
4. contrary	8. semifinal	

5 A Look Back

1. The setting is in the country because Shakespeare mentions the shepherd, a pail of milk, and brooding birds.

2. Any two of the following: icicles hanging, bearing logs, wind blowing, coughing drowning the parson's saying, birds brooding, Marian's red, raw nose.
3. Any two of the following: the shepherd blowing his nail, milk frozen in the pail, greasy Joan stirring the pot, crab apples roasting.
4. Answers will vary.

Lesson 10

1 Understanding the Story

1. The story is set on the planet Venus sometime in the future.
2. On this day the sun is going to shine for the first time in seven years.
3. Accept any of the following or similar details: Margot is different from the other children. She wouldn't play games with them. She would sing only about the sun. She remembered the sun from when she lived on Earth. She might return to Earth and see the sun again.
4. She won't adapt or fit in with the others. She recognizes that she is different. She is withdrawn and unfriendly.
5. The other children lock Margot in a closet before the rain stops and don't let her out again until after it starts again, so she misses the two hours of sunshine.
6. They actually have only two hours.
7. At first they were spellbound by the silence and the sight of the sun. Then they rushed outside, and ran and played wildly.
8. They seem to feel bad because now they understand why she is so sad. They may feel ashamed or sorry they locked her in. They feel reluctant to face her.

2 What Do You Think?

Answers will vary. Accept reasonable responses.

3 Synonym Review

1. before	8. dispute	15. sever
2. tradition	9. conclusive	16. doubt
3. adhere	10. massive	17. elude
4. mortal	11. abstain	18. revive
5. embarked	12. ceaseless	19. swell
6. bargain	13. undertaking	20. perception
7. kidnap	14. repel	

4 Looking Backward

1. exposition	5. distinct	9. affix
2. proposed	6. defrauding	10. required
3. detained	7. ill-fated	
4. obtained	8. encountered	

5 The Days of Our Lives

Part A

1. T   2. T   3. ?   4. F   5. ?

Part B

Answers will vary.

Review: Lessons 1-10

1 Definitions

1. innovation	7. tremor	13. testimony
2. Pharaoh	8. mariner	14. deposition
3. apparatus	9. posterity	15. disruption
4. oracle	10. desecration	16. expedition
5. exposition	11. repercussion	
6. spectacle	12. specimen	

2 Vocabulary Review

1. b	5. d	9. b	13. c
2. c	6. a	10. c	14. c
3. a	7. c	11. b	15. a
4. b	8. a	12. b	16. d

3 Antonym Review

1. release	6. active	11. careless
2. heed	7. immobile	12. attract
3. inactive	8. incompetent	13. ordinary
4. spirited	9. simple	14. deny
5. calm	10. linger	15. desist

4 More Durations

1. re, pro, con	5. e, re, trans
2. in, e, de	6. ex, con, pro
3. de, con, ob	7. per, of, ex
4. de, re, non	8. re, un, de

5 Past, Present, and Future

1. thumb	7. longevity	13. nutty
2. Hitler	8. ewe	14. affirm
3. elephant	9. tooth	15. rooster
4. swarm	10. organism	16. moth
5. ketchup	11. Napoleon	17. outskirts
6. effort	12. icicle	18. route

Look not mournfully into the past. It comes not back again. Wisely improve the present. Go forth to meet the future without fear.

Lesson 11

1 Understanding the Reading

1. b	3. a	5. c	7. c	9. c
2. a	4. b	6. b	8. c	

2 What Do You Think?

1. Chief Seattle's statement supports "A Fable for Tomorrow" because he says that when we harm the environment we harm ourselves. He says that all things are connected and related, and that whatever happens to the earth, happens to man as well.

2. Answers will vary. Reasonable responses include: Many Americans use biodegradable products. They obey anti-litter laws. They fight against pollution. They tend gardens.

3. Answers will vary. Reasonable responses include: Many Americans use products which pollute the atmosphere or environment. They cut down trees without replanting. They pollute waters by dumping garbage or sewage into them. They litter public places.

4. Answers will vary. Accept reasonable responses.

3 What Is the Nobel Prize?

1. anniversary, distinction, economics, substantial, enrichment

2. distinguished, accumulated, massive, portion, estate

3. abundance, tragedy, fateful, capable, incident

4. indignant, rebuild, determinedly, reliable, minimize

5. dedicated, ambitions, ample, exertion, inevitable

6. precisely, patents, discredited, reclusive, sociable

4 Names in Nature

1. b	3. b	5. c	7. b	9. b
2. b	4. a	6. c	8. a	10. c

5 The Good Earth

Part A

1. T	3. F	5. ?	7. F	9. T
2. T	4. T	6. T	8. ?	10. T

Part B

1. R	3. N	5. N
2. R	4. R	6. N

Lesson 12

1 Understanding the Reading: Part 1

1. a	3. d	5. d	7. d	9. d
2. b	4. b	6. a	8. c	10. a

2 Understanding the Reading: Part 2

1. Any two of the following or similar answers: Man has developed new ways to raise food crops, machines that use stored energy, and ways to cure or prevent diseases. Man is able to change the environment to suit his needs and desires.

2. Reasonable responses include: Man has exploited the limited supplies of forest, minerals and energy resources. Man has destroyed animal and plant populations. Huge areas of forests have been destroyed. Man has polluted the environment. Fossil fuels are being used up.

3. Man has polluted the environment and is using up the store of fossil fuels, and our survival as a species is threatened as a result.

What do you think? Accept reasonable responses.

3 Synonyms and Antonyms

1. abundant, skimpy
2. intricate, simple
3. decompose, develop
4. dismiss, employ
5. vigorous, drowsy
6. harmony, strife
7. contaminate, purify
8. affirm, deny
9. ruthless, merciful
10. withered, thriving
11. radiant, dull
12. prosperous, needy

4 Charting Information

Herbivores	Carnivores	Omnivores
grasshoppers	crocodiles	bears
hippopotamuses	sharks	human beings

Scavengers	Parasites
buzzards	fleas
vultures	ticks

5 Spelling Check

1. patriot
2. rogue
3. immigrant
4. nonconformist
5. coroner
6. etymologist
7. physician
8. hypnotist
9. infielder
10. landlady
11. instructor
12. Pharaoh

The name of the British conservationist: Prince Philip

Lesson 13

1 Understanding the Reading

1. a. a deep narrow gully; a gorge
   b. a road or trail that follows a winding, zigzag course up a steep grade
   c. loose fragments formed by breaking up or wearing away rock
   d. a mixture of water and other material such as soil, rock, or sand

2. The setting is the Cascade Range of mountains in the western U.S.

3. A mining company is about to start mining copper there.

4. He is the leader of Friends of the Earth.

5. He is a mineral engineer.

6. Park used that example to show how mining could improve the economic standard of living of people in the area of the mine.

7. Both Brower and Park agree that the ruins and debris left from the mining operation are ugly and spoil the beauty of the area. They both feel it was wrong to leave such a mess.

8. Brower believes in the conservation of natural resources, in recycling resources, and even going without some things in order to conserve some resources for future generations. Park believes that it is essential to use minerals to maintain and improve people's standard of living.

What do you think? Answers will vary. Accept reasonable responses.

2 The Earth: A Cartoonist's Point of View

Reasonable responses include:

1. He would probably agree with the cartoonist's point that man pollutes his environment and destroys the beauty of nature.

2. He would probably also agree that man's littering of his environment with trash is objectionable.

3. Answers will vary.

3 Word Families

1. vigorous, vigor
2. prosperity, prosper, prosperous
3. consistency, consistently, consistent, inconsistent
4. emphasize, emphatic, emphasis
5. probability, improbable, probable
6. complicated, complicate, complication

4 America's Resources

1. Florida
2. Horseshoe
3. Ontario, Erie, Huron, Michigan, Superior
4. Hernando
5. Minnesota
6. South Dakota
7. 1872
8. Utah
9. Colorado
10. Arizona
11. Hawaii
12. William

5 Can You Crack the Code?

1. copper
2. gold
3. tin
4. iron
5. lead
6. mercury
7. silver
8. chromium
9. manganese
10. cobalt

Lesson 14

1 Understanding the Story

1. a
2. d
3. d
4. c
5. c
6. b
7. c
8. d
9. a
10. b

2 What Do You Think?

Answers will vary. Reasonable responses include:

1. T.J. is persistent in trying to achieve his dream. He works hard and sets a good example for the others. He has a strong sense of purpose. He has knowledge and experience in growing things. He has a strong desire to have land on which to grow something.

2. The boys like the idea of a secret project. It gives them something to work together on. The uniqueness of the idea appeals to them. The project captures their imagination.

3 Word Relationships

1. b	3. a	5. c	7. d	9. b
2. c	4. d	6. b	8. a	10. c

4 From the Earth

1. hemlock
2. buckwheat
3. spearmint
4. sunflower
5. foxglove
6. goldenrod
7. arrowroot
8. horseradish
9. pennyroyal
10. heartsease

5 If You Were a Writer...

1. Zeus
2. Ares
3. Athena
4. Hercules
5. Narcissus
6. Aphrodite
7. Atlas
8. Pandora
9. Midas
10. Apollo

Lesson 15

1 Understanding the Story

1. The gang wants to plant grass and trees. T.J. tells them it will take a while to grow trees, but he goes along with their idea of planting grass when he sees how much it means to them. He gets them to agree to a row of watermelons, though.

2. Blackie steps on the young grass. The others don't do anything, because they can see he feels bad about what he did.

3. They are picking out the kind of watermelon seeds to buy from a catalog.

4. The owner is angry at the boys for being on his roof and for hauling up the dirt and planting grass there. He believes the weight on the roof could cause it to sag.

5. At first T.J. fights back because he believes his rights are being violated. The other boys have had more experience with adult authority and know they can't win. They are willing to leave the grass for the owner's men to remove, but T.J. looks at the earth as his, and doesn't want the men to touch it.

6. T.J. and the boys clear the grass and earth from the roof themselves.

2 What Do You Think?

1. Answers will vary. Accept reasonable responses.

---

2. Reasonable responses to why T.J. ran away include: He was homesick. He wanted to go back to where he could plant and raise a crop. He had suffered a great disappointment. He had seen his work destroyed. Opinions on the second part of the question will vary.

3 Which Word Does Not Fit?

1. Atlas
2. traverse
3. Polynesian
4. dedication
5. abstain
6. switchback
7. humble
8. laurel
9. wriggle
10. waddle
11. bale
12. Nobel
13. confer
14. wither
15. forebode

4 Homonym Review

1. doe—dough
2. Rome—roam
3. prey—pray
4. burrow—burro
5. council—counsel
6. aisle—isle
7. load—lode
8. sew—sow
9. principle—principal
10. bale—bail

5 A Logic Problem

	Jones	Kelly	Lane	North	artichokes	asparagus	broccoli	cauliflower
Alan	N	N	Y	N	N	Y	N	N
Bess	N	Y	N	N	N	N	Y	N
Dennis	N	N	N	Y	Y	N	N	N
Lucy	Y	N	N	N	N	N	N	Y
artichokes	N	N	N	Y				
asparagus	N	N	Y	N				
broccoli	N	Y	N	N				
cauliflower	Y	N	N	N				

Lucy Jones planted cauliflower.

Bess Kelly planted broccoli.

Alan Lane planted asparagus.

Dennis North planted artichokes.

Review: Lessons 1-15

1 Definitions

1. malady
2. specter
3. terrain
4. vigor
5. bravado
6. anonymous
7. substantial
8. emphatic
9. vegetation
10. levy
11. sediment
12. resolve
13. capability
14. migrant
15. diagnosis
16. cache

2 Using Context Clues: Part 1

1. angler—alder
2. consistently—desecration
3. spirited—skyrocketed
4. parapet—pondered
5. dabble—economics
6. recalled—insulting
7. contribution—infinitely
8. Characterized—transmitted
9. principles—council

3 Using Context Clues: Part 2

1. c   3. a   5. c   7. c
2. a   4. b   6. a

4 Putting Sentences in Order

2, 1, 3

3, 1, 4, 2

3, 4, 1, 2

5 A Poet's Point of View

Reasonable responses include:

1. We have shut ourselves off from the natural world. We shield ourselves from direct contact with the outside world and know it only through what we are told and shown by the media.
2. Mankind will continue to grow more distant and separated from nature. We will continue to lose touch with the natural world by refusing to be concerned.
3. Answers will vary.

Lesson 16

1 Understanding the Reading

I. A. Open fireplace
   B. Fuel supply
   C. Tinderbox
   D. Coal furnace

II. A. Outhouse
   B. Baths
      1. Water
      2. Kitchens

III. A. Night log
   B. Curfew
   C. Water pitcher
   D. Bed warmer

2 What Do You Think?

1. Answers will vary. Accept reasonable responses.
2. Answers will vary.

3 Using Context Clues

1. All, nothing, endures
2. nature, trial, silly
3. constantly, consist, actually, believe
4. fact, pace, human
5. Wars, caused, institutions, organized
6. years, reverse, Refrain, matters
7. change, life, truths, favor
8. change, remain, same

4 Writing about Change

Answers will vary.

5 Inventors and Their Inventions

1. Robert Fulton
2. Eli Whitney
3. Samuel F. B. Morse
4. Charles Goodyear
5. Cyrus McCormick
6. Samuel Colt
7. Elias Howe
8. George Westinghouse
9. Alexander Graham Bell
10. Thomas Edison
11. George Eastman
12. William Burroughs
13. George W. Carver
14. Ransom E. Olds
15. Lee DeForest

Lesson 17

1 Understanding the Play

1. Stepan thinks that Ivan has come to borrow money.
2. Ivan intends to ask Natalia to marry him.
3. They begin to quarrel over the ownership of some meadowland.
4. Answers will vary. Students who believe that the argument pertains to trivial matters may cite Natalia's statement that "the meadows are worth very little" and Ivan's willingness to give them to her. Other students may feel that five acres worth "a few hundred roubles" would be a serious matter. Students may also cite Natalia's statement that it is "the injustice of the thing" and Ivan's being "concerned with the principle" as indicating that the argument pertains to serious matters.
5. First he offers to give the meadows to Natalia. Later he threatens to take the matter to court.
6. She finds out he had come to propose marriage to her.
7. Answers will vary. Reasonable responses include: His daughter is very changeable; first she is angry with Ivan, then she wants him back. It is difficult to get a grown daughter married and on her own.
8. The play is intended to be humorous. Supporting evidence will vary. Students may cite the exaggerated reactions of the characters, the foolishness of the argument, the fact that both Ivan and Natalia claim to be dying at the end, and similar examples as evidence.

2 You Be the Playwright

Answers will vary. The following is what actually happens. When Ivan returns, Natalia apologizes and tells him the meadows are really his. Then she tries to lead the conversation to a point where he will propose to her. Instead, another argument breaks out, this time about the relative worth of their hunting dogs. Stepan is again drawn into the fray. Finally Ivan faints. Natalia and Stepan think he is dead. But Ivan recovers and Stepan tells him that Natalia consents to his proposal (although Ivan hasn't actually proposed to her yet). Ivan and Natalia hesitantly express their mutual happiness, but they resume their argument as Stepan calls for champagne and the curtain falls.

3 More about Anton Chekhov

1. monotonously, monotony, monotonous
2. Uninspired, inspiration, inspired
3. severity, severely, severe
4. reliably, unreliable, reliability
5. wretchedly, wretchedness, wretched
6. irritate, irritable, irritation
7. censorship, censor, uncensored
8. immodest, modesty, modest
9. mortally, mortal, immortality, immortal

4 Synonym Review

1. danger	7. adaptable	13. difficult
2. foundation	8. climb	14. flutter
3. ponder	9. leaning	15. obvious
4. harvest	10. influence	16. flow
5. scheme	11. splendid	
6. pause	12. household	

5 Foreign Currency

1. dollar	6. drachma	11. guilder
2. yuan	7. rupee	12. peseta
3. krone	8. lira	13. pound
4. mark	9. yen	14. deutsche mark
5. franc	10. peso	

Lesson 18

1 Understanding the Reading

1. a	3. a	5. d	7. c
2. b	4. c	6. c	8. c

2 Optimists and Pessimists

Answers will vary. Reasonable responses include:

2. a. Human beings can choose to be happy and most of them will.
   b. Most people can't choose to be happy; too many things happen to make them unhappy.
3. a. I agree that most people can be trusted and are concerned and friendly.
   b. Most people really can't be trusted. They don't care about other people, and they're unfriendly.
4. a. A person is always free to use his mind and his free will, no matter where he is.
   b. Man is a prisoner of his fate and of the circumstances of his life.
5. a. I'll welcome change and adapt to changing circumstances because I know it will be for the best.
   b. Most of the time things change for the worst, so I resist change as much as possible.

3 Antonym Review

1. trusting	6. pleasant	11. refined
2. willful	7. foreign	12. security
3. praise	8. integrity	13. optimistic
4. disperse	9. commonplace	14. safe
5. unusual	10. observant	15. abstinence

4 Signs of Change

1. ecologist	5. navigator	9. missionary
2. psychologist	6. ambassador	10. economist
3. sociologist	7. mayor	
4. tutor	8. grocer	

5 An Inventor's Advice

KAYOS 2 OKAYS	LATER 23 ALERT	MONAD 25 NOMAD	SMALL 7 MALLS	EXIST 8 EXITS
TUTOR 4 TROUT	FIRED 16 FRIED	SLIDE 9 IDLES	YEMEN 14 ENEMY	PAGES 22 GAPES
CHASE 21 ACHES	NOBLE 11 NOBEL	SEVER 13 VERSE	MANOR 15 ROMAN	STRUT 5 TRUST
ZONED 20 DOZEN	LEASE 12 EASEL	DOORS 17 ODORS	REINS 10 SIREN	MITES 6 ITEMS
SETUP 18 UPSET	CURBS 3 SCRUB	ALLOY 1 LOYAL	RUNES 19 NURSE	TRINE 24 INERT

Benjamin Franklin's words of advice: Lost time is never found again.

Lesson 19

1 Understanding the Reading

1. Roy Campanella played for the Dodgers for 10 years and was voted Most Valuable Player of the Year three times during those 10 years.
2. On this date, Roy Campanella was in an automobile accident that left him paralyzed.
3. She told him how much his courage and his faith had inspired her when she was in the same hospital.
4. Campanella felt that he was lucky to have been able to play baseball for 20 years.
5. As great ceramics are only made by surviving the white heat of the kiln, so suffering can produce in people a strength and an understanding beyond that normally found.
6. Quadriplegics are a rugged breed because they have survived great suffering and have learned from it.

7. He supposedly wrote a poem that moved Roy Campanella very much.

8. Campanella believes that he is lucky to be alive and to have learned from his tragic experience.

2 What Do You Think?

1. Roy Campanella's accident marked the end or finish of his career as a major league baseball player. However, during his long struggle to recuperate, he set and reached new goals for himself regularly. The definition of *finis* as a goal is closer to his philosophy because he never gave up. He says, "I have made a great deal of progress. I'm going to make more." His new goal is to help others like himself who are severely handicapped.

2. Answers will vary.

3 The Invention of Baseball

1. team
2. bases
3. a. E - pitcher's mound
   b. A - home plate
   c. B - first base
   d. D - third base
4. apart (from each other)
5. In 1834, the pitcher was instructed to toss the ball gently. Pitchers today try to throw the ball as fast and as skillfully as they can.
6. Without the diagram it would be difficult to follow the description of the game. Also, the reader wouldn't realize that the bases have been reversed since the early days.
7. Students' responses should include the points which form the baseball diamond, i.e., home plate, first base, second base, and third base, plus the pitcher's mound and the catcher's box. Any other details, such as fielders' positions and foul lines, are acceptable.

4 Change: Another Type of Response

Reasonable responses include:

1. Roy Campanella stopped playing because he was paralyzed in an accident. Flick Webb stopped playing because he finished high school.
2. Roy accepted the change as a new challenge and went on striving to better himself and to find new meanings to life. Flick seemed to drift into a routine; he stopped trying to learn and lived mostly in the past.
3. Roy learned through suffering to value whatever life brings; he was determined not to give up. Flick apparently didn't try to find other ways to use his talents or to train himself to do other things.
4. Answers will vary. Accept reasonable responses.
5. Answers will vary.

5 Word Relationships

1. c	4. b	7. d	10. a
2. a	5. a	8. b	11. b
3. a	6. c	9. d	12. d

Lesson 20

1 Understanding the Reading

1. c	3. c	5. c	7. b
2. d	4. d	6. a	

2 Reacting to the Reading

Reasonable responses include:

1. People can gain new insights and understand the world better. They see the world around them differently and an older, wider world opens to them. People are able to develop a value system based on the experiences and wisdom of many people in the past. People can develop new habits and attitudes. They discover a background that is richer than any single family can provide.

2. Answers will vary. Accept reasonable responses.

3. To establish a link with the past one might: read the great classics of the past; study history, philosophy, anthropology; become acquainted with great works of art; visit museums; talk with older people and with those who have studied the past.

3 A Poem by Langston Hughes

1. a. A river in southwest Asia flowing from Turkey to the Persian Gulf
   b. A river of central Africa rising in Zaire and emptying into the Atlantic
   c. The world's longest river, rising in Burundi and emptying into the Mediterranean Sea at Egypt
   d. A city in southeast Louisiana near the mouth of the Mississippi River

Reasonable responses include:

2. Hughes says he has "known rivers ancient as the world," "bathed in the Euphrates when dawns were young," "raised the pyramids above" the Nile, and "heard the singing of the Mississippi when Abe Lincoln went down to New Orleans." His "soul has grown deep" by making these experiences of the human past his own.

3. Hughes compares rivers with the flow of blood in human veins, life lines that keep lands and people alive through the ages. Forests die and mountains wear away; both are stationary. But rivers flow on forever; always remaining, always changing.

4. If Hughes had said his mind had "grown deep" he would imply that only his thinking had been affected. Likewise saying his heart had "grown deep" would imply that only his feelings were involved. The concept of soul encompasses both the mind and the heart and implies that his whole spirit has been enriched by his learning.

4 Synonyms and Antonyms

1. obstacle, advantage	6. shielded, unprotected
2. ample, stingy	7. despise, admire
3. ignite, extinguish	8. leaning, unwillingness
4. rehabilitate, damage	9. corrupt, honorable
5. sentimental, unemotional	10. elevate, lower

5 Spelling Check

1. historical
2. expedition
3. celebrate
4. Pilgrims
5. fowl
6. all right
7. forty
8. according
9. all right
10. fourth
11. observance
12. thankful

Review: Lessons 1-20

1 Definitions

1. canopy
2. plight
3. flux
4. famine
5. decade
6. shoddy
7. palpitation
8. unabridged
9. infirmity
10. obstacle
11. precarious
12. savvy
13. potential
14. technology
15. interval
16. minority

2 Vocabulary Review

1. b
2. c
3. d
4. a
5. a
6. d
7. b
8. a

3 Vocabulary Review

1. abridged
2. portable
3. competitive
4. sentimental
5. economical
6. reliable
7. desolate
8. offensive

4 Growth and Change

1. Pertaining to country, farming, or agricultural areas
2. Pertaining to city areas or highly-populated areas
3. 1869
4. World War I
5. 1929
6. 1930-1959
7. 1960-1987
8. 242,599,900

5 Time and Change

1. teeter
2. ragweed
3. aspirin
4. nags
5. shoot
6. feast
7. oyster
8. remedy
9. modest
10. anxiety
11. typhoon
12. Iowa
13. October
14. niche

Yesterday is experience. Tomorrow is hope. Today is getting from one to the other as best we can.

The synonym for *change*: Transformation

Word Indexes for Book 8

Word Index: Lessons 1 - 5

A

able-bodied
accompaniment
accumulate
accurate
accurately
activist
admiration
admirer
adopt
advertiser
alarmist
amazingly
ambassador
ambition
ambulance
Americanization
ample
anthropologist
anthropology
appendix
Arabian
Arabic
archaeologist
archaeology
Arthur
aspect
assumption
astrology
attach
attentive
attraction
attractive
attractiveness
Austin
Australian
authority
awakening
award

B

ballet
bearable
bearing
Beatrice
beautify
Bess
bewilderment
biological
biology
blockhead
boastfully

bold-faced
bombardment
Borneo
boundless
braggart
Budapest

C

calling
capitalism
Capricorn
captive
changeless
Charleston
cheerless
chloroform
civilize
civilized
cleverly
collar
commercial
complexion
comprise
confirmation
conformist
context
continually
contraption
contrast
contribute
conviction
coral
corset
critic
criticism
cruelty
cutter
cynic
cynicism

D

darken
David
deception
defenseless
demonstration
derrick
designer
determinedly
disapprove
disentangle
dishonorable

dismember
dispute
distinction
distinguished
distribute
distribution
Dover
dramatist

E

ecologist
ecology
economy
edit
effectively
Ehrich
elderly
eliminate
elimination
embezzle
engrave
Englishman
enrichment
entry
environment
environmental
envision
equator
escapism
escapist
Eskimo
etymologist
etymology
eventually
evolution
exception
executive
exhibition
exotic
expectation
expensiveness
extricate
extrication

F

fabulous
fantasy
fascinate
fascination
fateful
favoritism
feat

fencer
fiction
fictional
fifth
Fiji
frill
fulfillment

G

gallows
geologist
geology
gesture
glaring
gloss
Godfrey
gradually
Guam
guardian

H

Haida
hangman
hateful
Hawaiian
headliner
Henri
Henry, O.
heroism
hesitatingly
hijack
historical
ho
Houdini
hover
humanity
humbly
humility
Hungarian
Hungary
hypnotism

I

idealism
idealistic
identification
ignorant
illusion
illusionist
imagery
imitate
imitation

immigrant
immigrate
immune
impel
impressive
imprint
imprisonment
inconvenient
indication
individualism
Indonesia
ingrain
initiation
insignificant
instinct
institute
Israel
italicized

J

jailbreak
Jean
Joel
journalist
justly

K

Kosinski, J.

L

laborer
latter
leisure
lighthearted
limitation
Long Island
loom
luxury

M

macintosh
majority
make-up
manual
manufacturer
marionette
Marshall
marvel
materialism
materialist
mayor
measurable
media

meek
meekly
Melanesia
memoirs
mesh
meteorologist
meteorology
mica
Micronesia
Midway
Milwaukee
minister
misrepresent
misrepresentation
missionary
modest
modestly
modesty
monotony
Montreal
motivate
mutilate

N

necessity
neutrality
New Guinea
newsworthy
nicotine
nineteenth
nomad
nonconformist
nonetheless
Norse
northeast
northwest
notion
novel
novelist

O

Oakland
objection
objective
obvious
obviously
occasionally
offensive
opposition
organism
originally
originate
overhear
overpower
override
owlet

P

paperback
parallel
pathology
patriotic
patriotism
penalty
pen name
perception
permanently
personally
petroleum
Pierre
Pittsburgh
pleadingly
policy
polka
Polynesia
Polynesian
portable
portrait
pretense
pretentious
primitive
printing
proportion
prosperity
psychology
publicity
publicize

Q

quantity
quibbler
quotation

R

reappear
rearrange
reasonable
reasonably
recipient
recognition
recurrent
red-hot
Red Sea
reef
relation
reliable
remarkably
reportedly
reproduce
reproduction
resemble
restraint
retain
robot

rogue
rugged
running
rupture

S

Sahara
salesmanship
secondary
seemingly
self-confidence
self-educated
self-portrait
separation
shabbiness
shackle
shamefulness
shone
shoot-out
showy
significant
similarity
skeptic
skeptical
skepticism
slowwitted
sociology
sporting
staleness
standing
stately
status
stingy
straitjacket
subjective
superiority
survival
sustain
Suva
symbolic
systematic

T

Tahiti
Tasmania
tattoo
technique
territory
terrorism
theology
thereof
Thompson
Tolstoy
Tonga
treadmill
trivia
trivial

tropic
tropical

U

unAmerican
unattractive
unbearable
unbiased
uncivilized
unconscious
unconvinced
undecided
undefined
undergarment
undergo
uneventful
universal
unmistakable
unprotected
unseal
unspoiled
unsuspecting
U.S.

V

valuable
variation
Veblen, T.
verb
Vietnam
visualize
vocabulary

W

wearer
Wilhelmina
will power
wondrous
workmanship
worldwide

X

X ray

Y

youthfulness

Z

zoology

Word Index: Lessons 6 - 10

A

abduct
absentee
abstain
abstract
accomplish
additional
adhere
adjoin
administer
affirm
affix
Agricola, G.
Albany
alien
anesthetic
anniversary
antibiotic
antidote
antimacassar
antiseptic
antisocial
apparatus
arc
arrival
aspirin
assassin
assertion
asterisk
astonishingly
astrologer
astrological
attain
Austrian
avalanche

B

bar mitzvah
battalion
battlefield
bedcover
Beverly Hills
biologist
blueness
boastfulness
boulder
boundary
Bridgeport
Britain
brontosaurus
bronze
Brutus
bullfrog
burial

Burns, G.
buzzard

C

Cairo
capable
Cassius
cathedral
Celt
certainty
Chatham
childlessness
chime
chlorine
circumference
circumstantial
circumvent
cluster
colonial
Como
compel
conception
conclusive
concur
conditioner
confer
congestion
conscience
conservation
continuity
contradict
contradiction
contradictory
coroner
cosmic
counsel
counteract
coyote
Croesus
curiosity
Cyrus

D

daytime
declaration
dedicate
definite
defraud
delivery
Delphi
demote
denote
denounce
depart
depose

deposition
desecrate
desecration
desist
detain
diagnose
Diana
dictator
dimension
dinosaur
disastrous
discredit
disorganized
dispel
disregard
disruption
distasteful
distort
doth
duration

E

earthly
effectiveness
efficient
Egyptian
eject
elapse
eleventh
Elmira
elude
embalm
embank
embark
embattle
emit
emperor
encrust
ensnare
enthusiasm
entrails
ere
eruption
essential
estimate
ewe
exceptional
exceptionally
excessive
exclamation
exclusive
exertion
expedition
exposition
expressive

extensive
extinct
extinction
Ezekiel

F

feverish
fiesta
Filipino
finite
footfall
footrace
Fordham
forebear
forebode
forefather
foreleg
foremost
forenoon
foresight
foretell
fossil
fossilize
Frigga
frightfulness

G

gatherer
genus
Geoffrey
geographic
geological
gigantic
Gobi
granger
grouping

H

Hartford
hasten
Havana
hawkweed
healer
hence
heritage
hind leg
hindsight
hippopotamus
hitchhike
horrify
houseguest
hydra

I

icicle
Ides
ill-advised
ill-fated
ill-gotten
ill-used
immobile
imposition
inactive
inclusive
incomparable
inconsistent
indefinite
indicator
indisputable
industrial
inefficient
inevitable
infinite
inhabit
inhabitant
innovation
instinctive
intermix
interpret
interpretation
intricate
intricately
Isaiah
ivory

J

Janus
Jeremiah
Johann
Julius Caesar

K

L

Laplander
learned
legality
lesser celandine
leveler
likelihood
limber
lizard
locality
logically
loner
longevity

Longfellow, H.
long-range
Lugosi, B.

M

mallard
mammoth
Manila
Margot
mariner
martini
massive
memorabilia
merit
Merlin
Mesozoic
microsecond
migration
milestone
millionth
millisecond
minimize
misconception
misgiving
mislead
misled
mismanage
mobile
Mohammedanism
Monmouth
Moses
moss
muffle
mutilation

N

nanosecond
Napoleon
nasturtium
nationality
navigate
negotiate
negotiation
Nellie
New Haven
Niagara Falls
nightly
nomadic
Norah
norm
Norwalk
Nostradamus
notochord

O

observance
octopi

Odin
Old Testament
oracle
overdo
overpopulation
overslept

P

painstaking
particles
penicillin
perish
perishable
permissible
permissive
perpetual
Persia
Persian
Pharaoh
philosophic
phylum
platypus
portion
posterior
posterity
postmortem
postpone
postscript
posture
preside
prevail
prickly
priestess
priestly
primrose
profess
propel
provoke
psychologist
publication
purify
pyramid

Q

R

radius
raindrop
readjust
rearview
reassure
reclusive
recognizable
recur
reestablish
regulator
reinforce

relaxation
remedy
repel
repercussion
reputation
reread
resilient
resuscitate
retort
rodlike
Roosevelt
Ross, B.

S

sacred
sandstorm
Sarah
sauropod
savor
Scandinavian
scavenger
Schiller, J.
seasonal
seer
self-contempt
self-discipline
semicircle
semifinal
semiformal
semiprecious
sever
sew
Shakespeare, W.
shipping
siesta
significance
significantly
simplify
skyward
sociable
sofa
solemn
soothsayer
Spaniard
specimen
spectacle
spirited
squint
stagnant
statesman
stopwatch
stumpy
subdivide
subsist
sundrop
supercharge

superduper
superficial
surge
surprisingly
suspend
swarm
swindle
synchronize

T

tangerine
tatting
testimony
thinness
tidal
timekeeping
Titanic
trackway
transcribe
transfix
transgress
transistor
tremendously
tremor
tumultuously
turbulence
Tyr
Tyrannosaurus

U

underpart
undertaken
undertaking
undeserved
undoubtedly
ungodly
uninjured
unparalleled
unreal
unreliable
untangle
uproot
uptight
U.S.S.R.
utility

V

Valhalla
Vancouver
varied
venture
vertebra
vertebrate
vigorous
vital
volcanic

W

wakefulness
warmness
Waterloo
weather-beaten
Wells, H. G.
Westinghouse
wickerwork
Williamsport
Woden

X

Y

yellowness

Z

Word Index: Lessons 11 - 15

A
abandon
abundance
abundant
accessible
aftermath
Alan
alder
alligator
angler
anonymous
Antaeus
antelope
Arcadia
areaway
arrowroot
artichoke
asparagus
athletically
Atlas
Australasia

B
bale
befall
Berkeley
bestrewn
biologically
birdseed
bison
Black Hills
Borlaug, N.
brackish
bravado
Brazil
Brazilian
broccoli
Brower, D.
buckwheat

C
cache
canyon
capability
capacity
carnivore
Carson City
Carson, R.
cascade
catalogue
cauliflower
Choctaw
clod
cobalt

combatant
competition
complicate
complicated
complication
condone
conservationist
consistency
consistent
consistently
consolation
constructive
contaminate
contamination
contemplate
contemplation
contention
contribution
conversationally
corrugated
corruption
council
counselor
counterpart
cowardice
crabgrass
crater
crinkle

D
dabble
DDT
decompose
decomposer
dedication
deface
definitely
dejectedly
delta
de Soto, H.
detritus
diagnosis
digitalis
dilate
dispenser
distracted
distraction
doll
domain
dusky

E
ecologically
economics
ecosystem

efficiently
elementary
emphasize
emphatic
enormous
enterprise
environmentalist
Ernst
erosion
esoteric
estuary
excel
exploit

F
favorable
fearsome
filling
finality
fishery
fling
foreboding
foreground
foxglove
frenzied
freshwater

G
Gila monster
glen
god-awful
goldenrod
Grand Canyon
granular
Great Lakes
greenness
gruffly

H
habitat
Haeckel, E.
hare
harmony
harshness
hay fever
heartsease
heating
hemlock
herbivore
Hercules
Hernando
hesitant
honeycomb
horseradish

housefly
housekeeping
Howe
hydraulic

I
illustrate
immorally
improbable
inaction
independently
indiscriminately
inevitably
infielder
infinitely
ingredient
initial
integrity
intently
interior
international

J
jealousy

K
Kansas City
Kennecott

L
laborious
laboriously
laurel
lethal
levy
literature
lode
long-term
Louisiana

M
macabre
malady
malaria
malnourished
manganese
manipulation
marine
Marine
Marion
materially
Mauna Loa
maximum
Maxwell

McKinley, W.
McPhee, J.
melon
Mesabi Range
Mexico City
microorganism
migrant
Minas Gerais
mineral
mineralogy
Montana
moribund
mosquito
Mount McKinley
muskrat
mustang
mythical

N
nakedness
Narcissus
New Orleans
niche
Nobel, A.

O
omnivore
Ontario
ore
ornament
overstretch

P
Painted Desert
pallbearer
Pandora
parapet
parasite
parental
parentheses
parsley
patriot
peashooter
penalize
pennyroyal
percentage
pesticide
peter
piping
plaque
pocketful
poison ivy
poison oak
pollination

pollution
ponder
postwar
potent
potential
Powell, J. W.
precedence
predation
predator
prey
principle
probability
prosperous

Q

quicksilver

R

Rachel
radiant
radiation
radish
ragweed
rapidly
ravine
recommend
repellent
reprint
resolve
resolute
restrict
Ribicoff, A.
richness
rightness
robust
rooftop
roundly
rumple
ruthless

S

sagebrush
sedan
sediment
selfishly
self-mastery
Seminole
shapely
shingle
showcase
sicken
sickly
Sierra
Sioux
situate
skyrocket
slurry

solidly
sow
specifically
specter
sterile
sterility
Stewart
stolid
subcommittee
substantial
substitute
succulent
Suiattle
surrender
switchback

T

tableware
Taft
tailing
tarantula
teeter
tenant
terrain
texture
toilsome
totter
toxic
trample
transcendent
traverse
tumbleweed

U

Udall, S.
uncomplicated
uncontrollable
unique
universally
unknowing
unmercifully
unnoticed

V

vacant
vegetate
vegetation
ventilator
viburnum
vigor
vigorously
violation
volcano

W

wartime
weatherman

wetland
wither
withheld
Woods Hole
worriedly

X

Y

yellow jacket
Yellowstone
yellowthroat
youthful

Z

Word Index: Lessons 16 - 20

A
Abe
ablaze
Abner
abstinence
accustom
adaptable
adoption
advanced
alloy
aloneness
Alonzo
amateur
Anton
anxiety
architect
arduous
ascend
assembly
assuredly
asunder

B
bah
ballplayer
bankrupt
barrier
basis
bathwater
bed warmer
Benjamin
berth
blatant
bosom
builder
Burroughs, W.

C
Campanella, R.
canopy
centralize
ceramics
chamber
Chekhov, A.
Clermont
clinker
Co.
coachman
Colt, S.
compensate
competitive
completeness
confederate
congregation
consciously
continual
corporation
corrupt
crisscross
currency

D
darkly
dead-end
decade
DeForest, L.
departure
desolate
despise
detour
deutsche mark
dipsomaniac
disciplinarian
dishonor
disruptive
dissatisfaction
dissatisfied
distinguish
distortion
Dodgers
domestic
Doubleday, A.
drachma
dumbfounded

E
East Germany
Eastman, G.
East River
economic
economical
economist
educator
electronic
electronics
elegance
elegant
elevate
Eli
Elias
embezzlement
equality
essentially
Euphrates
evaluate
exaggerate
extensively
external
extinguish

F
famine
farm hand
fatten
favorably
festivity
figment
flawless
flexible
flux
focus
footstool
foot warmer
franc
Frost, R.
Fulton, R.
furnishing

G
gadget
glutton
gluttony
Goodyear, C.
gorgeously
grocer

H
hammock
hath
hazard
hazardous
hearth
heir
heirship
Heraclitus
Hindu
historian
honorable
horizontally
householder
Howe, E.
Hughes, L.

I
ignition
illumination
illumine
immature
immersion
immodest
inattentive
incidentally
infirmity
inflexible
inherit
initially
inquiry
insufficient
integration
internal
interruption
interval
intrigue
intriguer
involuntary
irregularly
irritable
irritation
irritate
Ivan

J
Johnson, G. W.

K
Karr, A.
kayo
kiln
kinship
krone

L
layman
leaning
librarian
lira
long-distance
lovesick
lower-class
lull
luncheonette

M
magnify
manor
materialistic
meditate
Menlo Park
Mexican
middle-class
minority
mite
monad
monotonous
monotonously
morrow
Morse, S.
mortally
motivation

N
Natalia
naught
navigator
negativity
neglect
Nehru, J.
Netherlands
Newfoundland
nightcap
nightshirt

O
oaken
observant
obstacle
occupant
Olds, R.
optimist
organizer
outing
overshadow

P
palpitate
palpitation
Papa
paraplegic
participant
peculiar
perfection
pertain
peseta
pessimist
pessimistic
pinball
Plato
plight
plumbing
politics
porcelain
postponement
potter
precarious
predictable
prestige
proclamation
prone

Q
quad
quadriplegic

R

ratio
reap
recurrence
rehabilitation
rehabilitate
reinforcement
relearn
reliability
reliance
relive
replenish
richly
ridgepole
riveted
roadblock
rune
rupee

S

Samuel
satin
savvy
scoff
self-confident
self-made
sentimental
severity
sewer
shoddy
shortage
shuck
siren
sitz bath
sizable
snort
sociologist
so-so
Southeast Asia
spinal
spontaneous
subconscious
subconsciously
successive
suction
sufficient
sunup
suspicion
suspicious

T

technologist
technology
telegraph
telegraphy
tendency
terribly

tester
thermostat
tinderbox
'tis
trine
tuberculosis
tutor

U

ugh
unabridged
uncensored
underestimate
unemotional
uninspired
United Kingdom
unlearn
unplanned
unpleasantness
unprincipled
unreasonable
unspoken
unyielding
Updike, J.
uplift
uprightness

V

verbally
Vero Beach
Vinson, F. M.
voluntarily
voluntary
vulgar

W

wafer
wagonload
washstand
West Germany
wheatland
Whitney, E.
wholeheartedly
willfully
workable
worthwhile
wretchedness
wrought

X

Y

Yemen
yen
yuan

Z

Word Index: Lessons 1 - 20

A

abandon
abduct
Abe
ablaze
able-bodied
Abner
absentee
abstain
abstinence
abstract
abundance
abundant
accessible
accompaniment
accomplish
accumulate
accurate
accurately
accustom
activist
adaptable
additional
adhere
adjoin
administer
admiration
admirer
adopt
adoption
advanced
advertiser
affirm
affix
aftermath
Agricola, G.
Alan
alarmist
Albany
alder
alien
alligator
alloy
aloneness
Alonzo
amateur
amazingly
ambassador
ambition
ambulance
Americanization
ample
anesthetic
angler
anniversary

anonymous
Antaeus
antelope
anthropologist
anthropology
antibiotic
antidote
antimacassar
antiseptic
antisocial
Anton
anxiety
apparatus
appendix
Arabian
Arabic
arc
Arcadia
archaeologist
archaeology
architect
arduous
areaway
arrival
arrowroot
Arthur
artichoke
ascend
asparagus
aspect
aspirin
assassin
assembly
assertion
assumption
assuredly
asterisk
astonishingly
astrologer
astrological
astrology
asunder
athletically
Atlas
attach
attain
attentive
attraction
attractive
attractiveness
Austin
Australasia
Australian
Austrian
authority

avalanche
awakening
award

B

bah
bale
ballet
ballplayer
bankrupt
bar mitzvah
barrier
basis
bathwater
battalion
battlefield
bearable
bearing
Beatrice
beautify
bedcover
bed warmer
befall
Benjamin
Berkeley
berth
Bess
bestrewn
Beverly Hills
bewilderment
biological
biologically
biologist
biology
birdseed
bison
Black Hills
blatant
blockhead
blueness
boastfully
boastfulness
bold-faced
bombardment
Borlaug, N.
Borneo
bosom
boulder
boundary
boundless
brackish
braggart
bravado
Brazil
Brazilian

Bridgeport
Britain
broccoli
brontosaurus
bronze
Brower, D.
Brutus
buckwheat
Budapest
builder
bullfrog
burial
Burns, G.
Burroughs, W.
buzzard

C

cache
Cairo
calling
Campanella, R.
canopy
canyon
capability
capable
capacity
capitalism
Capricorn
captive
carnivore
Carson City
Carson, R.
cascade
Cassius
catalogue
cathedral
cauliflower
Celt
centralize
ceramics
certainty
chamber
changeless
Charleston
Chatham
cheerless
Chekhov, A.
childlessness
chime
chlorine
chloroform
Choctaw
circumference
circumstantial
circumvent

civilize
civilized
Clermont
cleverly
clinker
clod
cluster
Co.
coachman
cobalt
collar
colonial
Colt, S.
combatant
commercial
Como
compel
compensate
competition
competitive
completeness
complexion
complicate
complicated
complication
comprise
conception
conclusive
concur
conditioner
condone
confederate
confer
confirmation
conformist
congestion
congregation
conscience
consciously
conservation
conservationist
consistency
consistent
consistently
consolation
constructive
contaminate
contamination
contemplate
contemplation
contention
context
continual
continually
continuity

contradict
contradiction
contradictory
contraption
contrast
contribute
contribution
conversationally
conviction
coral
coroner
corporation
corrugated
corrupt
corruption
corset
cosmic
council
counsel
counselor
counteract
counterpart
cowardice
coyote
crabgrass
crater
crinkle
crisscross
critic
criticism
Croesus
cruelty
curiosity
currency
cutter
cynic
cynicism
Cyrus

D

dabble
darken
darkly
David
daytime
DDT
dead-end
decade
deception
declaration
decompose
decomposer
dedicate
dedication
deface
defenseless
definite

definitely
DeForest, L.
defraud
dejectedly
delivery
Delphi
delta
demonstration
demote
denote
denounce
depart
departure
depose
deposition
derrick
desecrate
desecration
designer
desist
desolate
de Soto, H.
despise
detain
determinedly
detour
detritus
deutsche mark
diagnose
diagnosis
Diana
dictator
digitalis
dilate
dimension
dinosaur
dipsomaniac
disapprove
disastrous
disciplinarian
discredit
disentangle
dishonor
dishonorable
dismember
disorganized
dispel
dispenser
dispute
disregard
disruption
disruptive
dissatisfaction
dissatisfied
distasteful
distinction
distinguish

distinguished
distort
distortion
distracted
distraction
distribute
distribution
Dodgers
doll
domain
domestic
doth
Doubleday, A.
Dover
drachma
dramatist
dumbfounded
duration
dusky

E

earthly
East Germany
East River
Eastman,G.
ecologically
ecologist
ecology
economic
economical
economics
economist
economy
ecosystem
edit
educator
effectively
effectiveness
efficient
efficiently
Egyptian
Ehrich
eject
elapse
elderly
electronic
electronics
elegance
elegant
elementary
elevate
eleventh
Eli
Elias
eliminate
elimination
Elmira

elude
embalm
embank
embark
embattle
embezzle
embezzlement
emit
emperor
emphasize
emphatic
encrust
Englishman
engrave
enormous
enrichment
ensnare
enterprise
enthusiasm
entrails
entry
environment
environmental
environmentalist
envision
equality
equator
ere
Ernst
erosion
eruption
escapism
escapist
Eskimo
esoteric
essential
essentially
estimate
estuary
etymologist
etymology
Euphrates
evaluate
eventually
evolution
ewe
exaggerate
excel
exception
exceptional
exceptionally
excessive
exclamation
exclusive
executive
exertion
exhibition

exotic
expectation
expedition
expensiveness
exploit
exposition
expressive
extensive
extensively
external
extinct
extinction
extinguish
extricate
extrication
Ezekiel

F

fabulous
famine
fantasy
farm hand
fascinate
fascination
fateful
fatten
favorable
favorably
favoritism
fearsome
feat
fencer
festivity
feverish
fiction
fictional
fiesta
fifth
figment
Fiji
Filipino
filling
finality
finite
fishery
flawless
flexible
fling
flux
focus
footfall
footrace
footstool
foot warmer
Fordham
forebear
forebode

foreboding
forefather
foreground
foreleg
foremost
forenoon
foresight
foretell
fossil
fossilize
foxglove
franc
frenzied
freshwater
Frigga
frightfulness
frill
Frost, R.
fulfillment
Fulton, R.
furnishing

G

gadget
gallows
gatherer
genus
Geoffrey
geographic
geological
geologist
geology
gesture
gigantic
Gila monster
glaring
glen
gloss
glutton
gluttony
Gobi
god-awful
Godfrey
goldenrod
Goodyear, C.
gorgeously
gradually
Grand Canyon
granger
granular
Great Lakes
greenness
grocer
grouping
gruffly
Guam
guardian

H

habitat
Haeckel, E.
Haida
hammock
hangman
hare
harmony
harshness
Hartford
hasten
hateful
hath
Havana
Hawaiian
hawkweed
hay fever
hazard
hazardous
headliner
healer
hearth
heartsease
heating
heir
heirship
hemlock
hence
Henri
Henry, O.
Heraclitus
herbivore
Hercules
heritage
Hernando
heroism
hesitant
hesitatingly
hijack
hind leg
hindsight
Hindu
hippopotamus
historian
historical
hitchhike
ho
honeycomb
honorable
horizontally
horrify
horseradish
Houdini
housefly
houseguest
householder
housekeeping

hover
Howe
Howe, E.
Hughes, L.
humanity
humbly
humility
Hungarian
Hungary
hydra
hydraulic
hypnotism

I

icicle
idealism
idealistic
identification
Ides
ignition
ignorant
ill-advised
ill-fated
ill-gotten
illumination
illumine
ill-used
illusion
illusionist
illustrate
imagery
imitate
imitation
immature
immersion
immigrant
immigrate
immobile
immodest
immorally
immune
impel
imposition
impressive
imprint
imprisonment
improbable
inaction
inactive
inattentive
incidentally
inclusive
incomparable
inconsistent
inconvenient
indefinite
independently

indication
indicator
indiscriminately
indisputable
individualism
Indonesia
industrial
inefficient
inevitable
inevitably
infielder
infinite
infinitely
infirmity
inflexible
ingrain
ingredient
inhabit
inhabitant
inherit
initial
initially
initiation
innovation
inquiry
insignificant
instinct
instinctive
institute
insufficient
integration
integrity
intently
interior
intermix
internal
international
interpret
interpretation
interruption
interval
intricate
intricately
intrigue
intriguer
involuntary
irregularly
irritable
irritation
irritate
Isaiah
Israel
italicized
Ivan
ivory

J

jailbreak
Janus
jealousy
Jean
Jeremiah
Joel
Johann
Johnson, G. W.
journalist
Julius Caesar
justly

K

Kansas City
Karr, A.
kayo
Kennecott
kiln
kinship
Kosinski, J.
krone

L

laborer
laborious
laboriously
Laplander
latter
laurel
layman
leaning
learned
legality
leisure
lesser celandine
lethal
leveler
levy
librarian
lighthearted
likelihood
limber
limitation
lira
literature
lizard
locality
lode
logically
loner
long-distance
longevity
Longfellow, H.
Long Island
long-range
long-term

loom
Louisiana
lovesick
lower-class
Lugosi, B.
lull
luncheonette
luxury

M

macabre
macintosh
magnify
majority
make-up
malady
malaria
mallard
malnourished
mammoth
manganese
Manila
manipulation
manor
manual
manufacturer
Margot
marine
Marine
mariner
Marion
marionette
Marshall
martini
marvel
massive
materialism
materialist
materialistic
materially
Mauna Loa
maximum
Maxwell
mayor
McKinley, W.
McPhee, J.
measurable
media
meditate
meek
meekly
Melanesia
melon
memoirs
memorabilia
Menlo Park
merit

Merlin
Mesabi Range
mesh
Mesozoic
meteorologist
meteorology
Mexican
Mexico City
mica
Micronesia
microorganism
microsecond
middle-class
Midway
migrant
migration
milestone
millionth
millisecond
Milwaukee
Minas Gerais
mineral
mineralogy
minimize
minister
minority
misconception
misgiving
mislead
misled
mismanage
misrepresent
misrepresentation
missionary
mite
mobile
modest
modestly
modesty
Mohammedanism
monad
Monmouth
monotonous
monotonously
monotony
Montana
Montreal
moribund
morrow
Morse, S.
mortally
Moses
mosquito
moss
motivate
motivation
Mount McKinley

muffle
muskrat
mustang
mutilate
mutilation
mythical

N

nakedness
nanosecond
Napoleon
Narcissus
nasturtium
Natalia
nationality
naught
navigate
navigator
necessity
negativity
neglect
negotiate
negotiation
Nehru, J.
Nellie
Netherlands
neutrality
Newfoundland
New Guinea
New Haven
New Orleans
newsworthy
Niagara Falls
niche
nicotine
nightcap
nightly
nightshirt
nineteenth
Nobel, A.
nomad
nomadic
nonconformist
nonetheless
Norah
norm
Norse
northeast
northwest
Norwalk
Nostradamus
notion
notochord
novel
novelist

O

oaken
Oakland

objection
objective
observance
observant
obstacle
obvious
obviously
occasionally
occupant
octopi
Odin
offensive
Olds, R.
Old Testament
omnivore
Ontario
opposition
optimist
oracle
ore
organism
organizer
originally
originate
ornament
outing
overdo
overhear
overpopulation
overpower
override
overshadow
overslept
overstretch
owlet

P

painstaking
Painted Desert
pallbearer
palpitate
palpitation
Pandora
Papa
paperback
parallel
parapet
paraplegic
parasite
parental
parentheses
parsley
participant
particles
pathology
patriot
patriotic

patriotism
peashooter
peculiar
penalize
penalty
penicillin
pen name
pennyroyal
percentage
perception
perfection
perish
perishable
permanently
permissible
permissive
perpetual
Persia
Persian
personally
pertain
peseta
pessimist
pessimistic
pesticide
peter
petroleum
Pharaoh
philosophic
phylum
Pierre
pinball
piping
Pittsburgh
plaque
Plato
platypus
pleadingly
plight
plumbing
pocketful
poison ivy
poison oak
policy
politics
polka
pollination
pollution
Polynesia
Polynesian
ponder
porcelain
portable
portion
portrait
posterior
posterity

postmortem
postpone
postponement
postscript
posture
postwar
potent
potential
potter
Powell, J. W.
precarious
precedence
predation
predator
predictable
preside
prestige
pretense
pretentious
prevail
prey
prickly
priestess
priestly
primitive
primrose
principle
printing
probability
proclamation
profess
prone
propel
proportion
prosperity
prosperous
provoke
psychologist
psychology
publication
publicity
publicize
purify
pyramid

Q

quad
quadriplegic
quantity
quibbler
quicksilver
quotation

R

Rachel
radiant
radiation

radish
radius
ragweed
raindrop
rapidly
ratio
ravine
readjust
reap
reappear
rearrange
rearview
reasonable
reasonably
reassure
recipient
reclusive
recognition
recognizable
recommend
recur
recurrence
recurrent
red-hot
Red Sea
reef
reestablish
regulator
rehabilitate
rehabilitation
reinforce
reinforcement
relation
relaxation
relearn
reliability
reliable
reliance
relive
remarkably
remedy
repel
repellent
repercussion
replenish
reportedly
reprint
reproduce
reproduction
reputation
reread
resemble
resilient
resolute
resolve
restraint
restrict

resuscitate
retain
retort
Ribicoff, A.
richly
richness
ridgepole
rightness
riveted
roadblock
robot
robust
rodlike
rogue
rooftop
Roosevelt
Ross, B.
roundly
rugged
rumple
rune
running
rupee
rupture
ruthless

S

sacred
sagebrush
Sahara
salesmanship
Samuel
sandstorm
Sarah
satin
sauropod
savor
savvy
Scandinavian
scavenger
Schiller, J.
scoff
seasonal
secondary
sedan
sediment
seemingly
seer
self-confidence
self-confident
self-contempt
self-discipline
self-educated
selfishly
self-made
self-mastery
self-portrait

semicircle
semifinal
semiformal
Seminole
semiprecious
sentimental
separation
sever
severity
sew
sewer
shabbiness
shackle
Shakespeare, W.
shamefulness
shapely
shingle
shipping
shoddy
shone
shoot-out
shortage
showcase
showy
shuck
sicken
sickly
Sierra
siesta
significance
significant
significantly
similarity
simplify
Sioux
siren
situate
sitz bath
sizable
skeptic
skeptical
skepticism
skyrocket
skyward
slowwitted
slurry
snort
sociable
sociologist
sociology
sofa
solemn
solidly
soothsayer
so-so
Southeast Asia
sow

Spaniard
specifically
specimen
spectacle
specter
spinal
spirited
spontaneous
sporting
squint
stagnant
staleness
standing
stately
statesman
status
sterile
sterility
Stewart
stingy
stolid
stopwatch
straitjacket
stumpy
subcommittee
subconscious
subconsciously
subdivide
subjective
subsist
substantial
substitute
successive
succulent
suction
sufficient
Suiattle
sundrop
sunup
supercharge
superduper
superficial
superiority
surge
surprisingly
surrender
survival
suspend
suspicion
suspicious
sustain
Suva
swarm
swindle
switchback

symbolic
synchronize
systematic

T

tableware
Taft
Tahiti
tailing
tangerine
tarantula
Tasmania
tatting
tattoo
technique
technologist
technology
teeter
telegraph
telegraphy
tenant
tendency
terrain
terribly
territory
terrorism
tester
testimony
texture
theology
thereof
thermostat
thinness
Thompson
tidal
timekeeping
tinderbox
'tis
Titanic
toilsome
Tolstoy
Tonga
totter
toxic
trackway
trample
transcendent
transcribe
transfix
transgress
transistor
traverse
treadmill
tremendously
tremor
trine
trivia

trivial
tropic
tropical
tuberculosis
tumbleweed
tumultuously
turbulence
tutor
Tyr
Tyrannosaurus

U

Udall, S.
ugh
unabridged
unAmerican
unattractive
unbearable
unbiased
uncensored
uncivilized
uncomplicated
unconscious
uncontrollable
unconvinced
undecided
undefined
underestimate
undergarment
undergo
underpart
undertaken
undertaking
undeserved
undoubtedly
unemotional
uneventful
ungodly
uninjured
uninspired
unique
United Kingdom
universal
universally
unknowing
unlearn
unmercifully
unmistakable
unnoticed
unparalleled
unplanned
unpleasantness
unprincipled
unprotected
unreal
unreasonable
unreliable

unseal
unspoiled
unspoken
unsuspecting
untangle
unyielding
Updike, J.
uplift
uprightness
uproot
uptight
U.S.
U.S.S.R.
utility

V

vacant
Valhalla
valuable
Vancouver
variation
varied
Veblen, T.
vegetate
vegetation
ventilator
venture
verb
verbally
Vero Beach
vertebra
vertebrate
viburnum
Vietnam
vigor
vigorous
vigorously
Vinson, F. M.
violation
visualize
vital
vocabulary
volcanic
volcano
voluntarily
voluntary
vulgar

W

wafer
wagonload
wakefulness
warmness
wartime
washstand
Waterloo
wearer

weather-beaten
weatherman
Wells, H. G.
West Germany
Westinghouse
wetland
wheatland
Whitney, E.
wholeheartedly
wickerwork
Wilhelmina
willfully
Williamsport
will power
wither
withheld
Woden
wondrous
Woods Hole
workable
workmanship
worldwide
worriedly
worthwhile
wretchedness
wrought

X

X ray

Y

yellow jacket
yellowness
Yellowstone
yellowthroat
Yemen
yen
youthful
youthfulness
yuan

Z

zoology